The London Lupus Centre, Book of Lupus:
A Patients' Guide

G. Hughes

The London Lupus Centre, Book of Lupus: A Patients' Guide

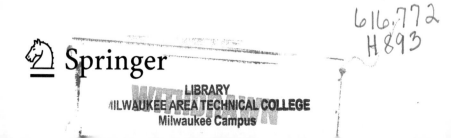

Springer

Graham Hughes
The London Lupus Centre
London Bridge Hospital
London, UK

ISBN 978-1-84800-373-6   e-ISBN 978-1-84800-374-3
DOI 10.1007/978-1-84800-374-3

British Library Cataloguing in Publication Data
A catalogue record for this book is available from the British Library

Library of Congress Control Number: 2008941264

Printed on acid-free paper

Springer Science+Business Media
springer.com

Contents

Preface

The London Lupus Centre at London Bridge Hospital opened two years ago. Staffed by a team of 8 consultants all of whom trained in the lupus unit at St Thomas' Hospital, and a support staff all experienced in lupus, the unit has two main aims:

- The first is to provide a clinical service for patients with lupus, Hughes syndrome and related conditions in an efficient and compassionate unit.

- The second, in collaboration with our three related charities – The St Thomas' Lupus Trust, The Hughes Syndrome Foundation, and Lupus UK – is to contribute to a greater awareness of these conditions both by the public and the medical nursing professions. This short volume is an attempt to do just that.

I am grateful to Sandy Hampson, Sharminy Ragunathan and Melanie Draper for their advice and help with the manuscript, and to Dr Christopher Edwards, one of the medical team at The London Lupus Centre for writing Chapters 15, 20, 24. Finally, I owe a debt to John Reay, CEO of London Bridge Hospital for his foresight in encouraging and supporting the setting up of our venture.

Graham Hughes
Head, London Lupus Centre
www.thelondonlupuscentre.co.uk

Lupus in a nutshell

Here is a summary of what is known (and what is not known) about lupus in 10 points:

1 **What is lupus?** Lupus is a disease in which the immune system becomes over-active. (Some have dubbed it the opposite of AIDS). This overactive immune system ends up producing too many antibodies, and potentially clogging up or damaging the delicate organs of the body (rather like a car using too rich a mixture of petrol or gasoline).

2 **Who gets lupus?** Most patients are young women, the peak age group being 15–50. Throughout the world the female:male ratio is 9:1.

3 **How common is lupus?** Approximately 1 in 1,000 women, though some estimates put the figure nearer 1 in 800. Thus lupus is more common, for example, than multiple sclerosis or leukaemia. The good news is that it is potentially treatable.

4 **Which countries are affected?** Lupus affects people from every country in the world. There have been reports that it may be more common in certain ethnic groups such as Afro-Caribbeans and in the Chinese.

5   **What causes lupus?** Nobody knows what kicks off the overactive immune system. Suspects include sunlight (UV light), hormones, stress, certain medicines and chemicals, and viruses. However, in many cases there is no clear culprit.

6   **Is it hereditary?** There is no doubt that some families have more than one member with lupus. In other families the genetic link is there, but less obvious (ie, other members of the family may have a related autoimmune condition, eg, a daughter with lupus, an aunt with thyroid disease, a grandmother with rheumatoid arthritis).

7   **How do I know if I have lupus?** The clinical features of lupus include fever, fatigue, rashes, aches and pains, and potentially life-threatening internal organ (kidney, heart, brain, etc) involvement. These are discussed in the next chapter and in more detail later in the book.

8   **What tests are there?** Most lupus patients can be diagnosed by a simple blood test. The doctor ticks 3 main boxes on the blood form – ANA, DNA and aCL (anti-cardiolipin). These are discussed in detail in Section 4.

9   **What treatments are available?** The spectrum of treatment for lupus patients has broadened in recent years. As well as a range of drugs, including antimalarials, steroids and immunosuppresives, treatment is also directed at lifestyle measures, management of related problems such as blood pressure, and prevention of conditions such as osteoporosis, thrombosis and coronary artery disease.

10 **The future?** The prognosis for lupus has improved out of all recognition. Once regarded as a 'doom and gloom, small print' disease, lupus is gaining recognition worldwide, with the majority of patients now able to lead a full and active life.

What to look for?

1 One of the difficulties for lupus patients is that the disease can show itself in a hundred different ways – indeed it is often called 'The Great Mimic'.

Key points

- Lupus is 'the great mimic'
- Symptoms include fatigue, rashes, hair loss
- Test for 'sticky blood'
- Most lupus pregnancies are uncomplicated

2 Clinical features of lupus – although lupus can present as an acute (flu-like) illness, more commonly it comes on gradually, often fluctuating in its severity. It is not uncommon, for example, for a woman diagnosed with lupus at the age of say 25, to have been having symptoms for at least 3 years.

3 Symptoms – the over-riding symptoms are fatigue, aches and pains, rashes, lack of energy. Headaches and gland swelling are common, indeed many lupus patients are initially diagnosed as having glandular fever.

4 Pre-lupus – it is not uncommon for lupus patients to give a history of vague symptoms going back to their teens, and even earlier. These include growing pains, headache and migraine (especially important in Hughes syndrome – see

Chapter 14), allergies (including insect bite allergies and allergies to antibiotics). A history of prolonged glandular fever (the Epstein–Barr virus) has been suspected as one of the causes of lupus.

5   Cold circulation – another feature which may pre-date the diagnosis by many years is cold circulation. This usually presents as Raynaud's phenomenon which is a tendency for the fingers (and often the toes) to turn white, then blue, sometimes leading to cold sores or chilblains.

6   Skin – rashes can occur on any part of the body. On the face, the most well known rash is the butterfly rash on the cheeks and nose. Hair loss can be an important feature of lupus, and a clue to diagnosis. In many cases but not all the skin rashes are made worse by UV light and some lupus patients are extremely sensitive to the sun.

7   Muscles and joints – rheumatic symptoms are common though, fortunately, rarely crippling. Often pains are more focused on the muscles or tendons.

8   Kidney – broadly speaking, inflammation of the kidneys is usually painless (silent) and picked up on urine and blood tests.

9   Brain – any one of the following brain symptoms can occur: headache, depression, phobias and seizures. This is a very important part of lupus and will be discussed later.

10   Heart and lungs – chest pain (usually pleurisy) is common during the acute phase of lupus. More serious heart involvement is rare, though as lupus patients are now living full and active lives, the focus on heart attack risk factors, such as raised cholesterol, is becoming increasingly important.

11   Clotting (Hughes syndrome) – in some lupus patients, there is a history of blood clots, such as deep vein thrombosis

(DVT). We can now identify this group of patients with simple blood tests. The 'sticky blood' syndrome, also known as the anti phospholipid syndrome or Hughes syndrome, is treatable and even preventable.

12 Pregnancy – for most lupus patients, pregnancy is uncomplicated. However, for a minority, problems can occur and monitoring is vital. This is especially so for those with Hughes syndrome, in whom clotting in the placenta can lead to recurrent miscarriage, although again this is largely preventable.

In summary, lupus can affect any part of the body, and the diagnosis can be missed. Furthermore, the up and down nature of the disease adds to the problem.

The main message for doctors and patients alike is to consider lupus as a potential diagnosis. The good news is that a simple blood test is usually sufficient to diagnose the condition, allowing treatment to be started in time to prevent serious organ damage.

The rise and rise of lupus

Lupus can, in many ways be considered a modern disease. Even as recently as 1970, lupus was considered rare. In the 1960s, the world map of lupus had huge empty spaces. It now seems remarkable that lupus was barely thought to exist in Africa, Australia, South America or China!

Key points

- Lupus is more common than multiple sclerosis
- Prevalence of 1 in 800 in some population groups
- Increasingly diagnosed world-wide
- New drugs becoming available

All that has changed dramatically. Lupus is now recognised in centres throughout the globe. The international journal LUPUS (http://lup.sagepub.com/) runs a regular feature called 'lupus around the world'. One of the messages from this series of articles is the broad similarity in the clinical features of lupus in different lupus clinics.

Ethnic differences

While the broad clinical picture of lupus is consistent, there may well be differences in the severity and frequency of lupus in different ethnic groups.

In the US, for example, lupus has long been considered more severe in Afro-Caribbean and Hispanic populations, with kidney disease and blood pressure being more common. In the UK, lupus may be more common in Asian and Afro-Caribbean populations, rising to 1 in 800 of women in these populations.

On of the big mysteries of lupus has been its apparent rarity in Africa. To some extent this may be because of missed diagnoses, however recent studies in London have shown that lupus is certainly emerging in African immigrants.

The history of lupus

The skin features of lupus, particularly the more disfiguring forms of discoid lupus, have been recognised for over two centuries. However, it was only in the late 19th century that a number of physicians, notably the great William Osler, painted a wider picture of the disease.

In 1948, recognition of the disease was given a great impetus with the discovery of a lupus blood test – the so-called LE cell test. This test is based on the observation that in lupus patients an abnormal or characteristic blood cell can be seen under the microscope.

Some years later, the more sensitive anti-nuclear antibody (ANA) test was developed and this test became the standard screening test for lupus.

The next major breakthrough in the late 1960s was the development of the anti-DNA test – a highly specific test for lupus. Finally, in 1983 the anti-cardiolipin test was developed, in parallel with a description of 'sticky blood' (or antiphospholipid) syndrome.

An early milestone in the treatment of lupus was the recognition in 1896 by Dr Thomas Payne of St Thomas' Hospital, London, that quinine could have a beneficial effect both on the fever and joint pains in lupus, as well as the skin rash.

In the 1940s Hench and his co-workers discovered the remarkable effects of steroids, lupus being one of the first diseases to benefit from this Nobel prize-winning discovery.

In the 1970s, the use of immunosuppressive drugs, notably pulse (intravenous) cyclophosphamide, was a major advance in the treatment of severe lupus, especially lupus nephritis.

Despite these advances, the list of drugs available for the treatment of lupus has remained disappointingly small, until recently. Now there are two new, promising drugs: mycophenolate (Cellcept®) and rituximab (Mabthera®).

Mycophenolate mofetil (MMF or Cellcept®) has been an extremely successful drug in the transplant world for many years and is already having a major impact in the treatment of lupus (see Chapter 21).

Rituximab is one of the family of monoclonals or designer drugs, having a specific action on the immune system's B cells (the cells responsible for the production of antibodies). Not only is this drug proving clinically useful, but the good news is that there are a number of similar agents in the pipeline.

Recent advances

What are the three major advances of recent times? Opinions will obviously differ – but here are mine:

1   The more conservative approach to treatment – reducing over-usage of steroids, and fine tuning of drugs such as cyclophosphamide.

2   The enormous improvement in prognosis – due not only to the direct treatment of the disease itself, but also paying attention to other related medical conditions such as high blood pressure, raised cholesterol and osteoporosis.

3 The impact of antiphospholipid syndrome on the management of lupus – many features previously thought to be due directly to lupus (eg, strokes, seizures, balance disorders, leg ulcers) are now known to be due to 'sticky' blood. This has meant, for many lupus patients, a treatment directed against the development of blood clots, rather than more and more steroids.

What causes lupus?

There is no known single cause of lupus. However, there are a number of well studied factors which undoubtedly contribute to the disease.

Key points
- Hereditary tendency
- Overactive immune system
- Influenced by hormones
- Possible environmental triggers

In simple terms, lupus is thought to be a condition with an inherited tendency for the immune system to go into overdrive. Some of the factors which are known to 'light the touch paper' include ultraviolet (UV) light, stress and hormone changes. A number of infectious as well as environmental factors are also suspected.

Genetics

Family and twin studies have shown convincingly that lupus has a hereditary tendency.

Lupus patients frequently have family histories of lupus, or of other autoimmune diseases. There are also numerous reports of large families with multiple cases of lupus.

Studies of twins with lupus are also interesting – the chance of an identical twin of a lupus patient developing the disease is 60%. For the geneticist, this figure suggests two things: firstly, that lupus has a definite genetic tendency and secondly, that this genetic predisposition is not the only factor in the disease (the twin statistic would be far higher in that case). Thus lupus is a disease of 'soil and seed' – genetics and environment.

The immune system in lupus

'A city where normal controls fail, law and order is poor, and the household rubbish lies on the street.' This, so the theory goes, is what happens in active lupus – the normal immune 'surveillance' breaks down, and the normal mechanism for removing cell 'waste' fails.

The normal, healthy immune system protects against foreign invaders such as viruses, bacteria or toxins by mounting what is called an 'immune response'. This response comes in two main forms – immune cells and protein antibodies. There are two main types of immune cells:

• T cells – the controlling or suppressor cells; and

• B cells – the worker cells which produce the antibodies.

In lupus there is an impaired suppressor response (loss of police control) and the worker B cells go into overdrive and produce excess antibodies. These antibodies can, in turn, cause damage to vital body parts such as the blood vessels and the blood cells.

More recently, a second and important defect has been found. The normal immune system not only neutralises invaders but plays an important part in 'rubbish clearance' – the removal of dead or damaged cells (the scientific term is apoptosis). Failure of this important role leads to a potentially damaging build up of unwanted material.

Much has been learnt about the ways in which the various cells in the immune system communicate with each other, and this knowledge has paved the way for a whole new generation of designer drugs.

In future, rather than giving immunosuppressives which are, sadly, capable of poisoning the good cells as well as the bad cells, drugs which specifically pinpoint certain cells will be the order of the day.

One such targeted treatment already showing great promise is rituximab (Mabthera®). This drug targets a specific marker (CD 20) on B cells and has a powerful effect on these antibody-producing cells.

Hormones

Why, in lupus clinics throughout the world, is the female:male ratio always 9:1? Why women?

Why does lupus flare pre-menstrually and, conversely, often stabilise at the time of the menopause?

It is clinically abundantly clear that sex hormones must play a part in the disease, and research has supported these observations. It is also known that these hormones (notably the female sex hormone oestrogen) can have a major impact on the working of the immune system. One obvious reason for this is pregnancy: the woman carries a fetus which by definition is half foreign; the pregnant woman's immune system must be able to deal with this to avoid rejection of the fetus.

Researchers have shown that oestrogen can, in lupus, heighten the immune response, while the male hormone testosterone has the opposite effect. Sadly, although many studies have been carried out, it has not been possible to convert this knowledge into clinical practice as yet.

The environment

Our lack of knowledge of the precise triggers in lupus has not stopped us building up a list of suspected environmental factors. These include viruses, sunlight, toxins and drugs, to name but a few, and will be discussed in the next chapter.

Lupus and the world around us

Why do I have lupus?

This common question is difficult to answer with certainty. However, in recent years we have increased our understanding of why someone develops lupus. It appears that the genes we inherit from our parents are responsible for some of the risk. In addition, the environment around us also plays an important role. Environmental factors that have been linked to lupus include exposure to sunlight, viruses and silica dust.

Different environmental factors may increase the risk of developing lupus. However, these will only be important in someone who may already have inherited lupus genes.

Key points

Triggering factors can include:

• UV light

• Stress

• Viral infections

Sunlight

Ultraviolet light that is present in sunlight can have two effects on lupus. Firstly, it can make lupus skin rashes worse. Secondly, it also appears to cause a more general flare of lupus in certain people. One piece of research work supporting this idea comes from Scandinavian countries that have a very big difference in seasonal exposure to sunlight. For example, people living near the Arctic Circle have summers that are light for nearly 24 hours per day and winters that are dark for nearly 24 hours per day. In these populations a lupus flare becomes more likely after sun exposure in the summer.

Smoking

Smoking has many negative effects on health. However, in recent years researchers have started to believe that smoking makes diseases like lupus and rheumatoid arthritis more severe. It may be that smoking stimulates the immune system to become more aggressive and begin the process that ends in lupus.

It is also very relevant that smoking impairs the beneficial effects of Plaquenil® (see p. 79).

Silica

Silica is a mineral that most people encounter as quartz on beaches or rocky outcrops. People who are exposed to silica dust, such as miners, stonemasons and sand blasters, are more likely to get lupus. The silica appears to stimulate the immune system. Clearly most people are not exposed to industrial silica dust, but perhaps lower levels may also produce some effects in certain individuals.

Viruses

Some common viruses have been linked to lupus. All of us are exposed to many different viruses during our lives. However, some individuals, perhaps those with the lupus genes, may over-react to them. The Epstein–Barr virus (EB) is responsible for causing infectious mononucleosis, more commonly known as glandular fever. There is increasing evidence that the EB virus may be one of the environmental factors that makes lupus more likely.

Lupus occurs when a patient's blend of genes, and environmental factors come together. Rather like being dealt a bad hand in a card game, it is not the individual card but the whole hand of cards that causes the problem. The world around us contains viruses, sunlight, dust, and many other factors. Some of these seem to be important in causing lupus to flare.

The clinical picture

The onset of lupus can be either dramatic (coming on over a period of days) or, more commonly, gradual (sometimes missed or wrongly diagnosed in its early stages).

> **Key points**
>
> Clinical features include:
>
> • Depression/headache
>
> • Cold circulation (Raynaud's)
>
> • Flu-like symptoms
>
> Lupus can settle down over time

Classical lupus

The most well known 'classical' picture of lupus is demonstrated by the following example.

A 22 year old woman with a 1–2 year history of vague general illness and fatigue develops fever, severe aches and pains, rashes, including a noticeable reddish rash on the cheeks and nose, and hair loss. Further testing reveals anaemia, a low white blood cell count and protein in the urine, suggesting kidney inflammation. Prior to this increase in symptoms, she may have gone through a particularly stressful period in her life (eg, at home or in college).

There is often, as in this clinical example, a suggestion that mild or 'grumbling' lupus had been present for months or even years before the diagnosis.

In this patient it is possible that stress contributed to the flare. While it is difficult to quantify stress, there is no doubt that this is a common story and one which does need more study.

However, while some triggering factors (eg, ultraviolet light, certain drugs such as Septrin®) are well recognised in lupus, in the majority of patients there is no clear antecedent history.

'Cold circulation' (Raynaud's)

Many lupus patients complain of cold fingers and toes. In some cases a more extreme form called Raynaud's phenomenon occurs, where the fingers (sometimes only one or two fingers) turn first white, then blue, and then red. In some patients (especially in children and teenagers), this 'cold circulation' can lead to small sores or chilblains on the tips of the fingers and toes. In many patients the history of cold circulation precedes the main diagnosis by many years.

It should be said that while Raynaud's phenomenon is troublesome to patients and in some cases severe, it rarely leads to more severe circulation disorders in lupus patients.

Fatigue

In any large survey of lupus, fatigue is the most common complaint. Often it is the sole and overwhelming symptom.

Aches and pains

High on the list of symptoms and often flu-like, the pains associated with lupus are not simply confined to the joints, but affect muscles and tendons, giving rise to the 'pain all over' description so often reported in active lupus. The joints can be swollen, but rarely to the degree seen in rheumatoid arthritis. Importantly, the joints seldom become permanently damaged, again unlike rheumatoid arthritis.

Tendon problems can be prominent; for example, the fingers can feel tight and bendy (difficulty saying one's prayers) and, in more severe cases, the fingers and thumb can become pulled out of shape. The 'hitch-hiking' thumb is an unusual but very characteristic feature in some lupus patients.

Rashes

Any rash can occur, though sun-exposed areas such as the face, the V of the neck, ear lobes and hands are especially frequently involved. The rashes are commonly worse after sun exposure.

Involvement of the scalp leads to hair loss, often mild, but sometimes patchy and even severe; this is an important clue in making a diagnosis.

Depression

This can be an important feature of lupus. It is often dismissed as merely secondary to the aches and pains of lupus. Wrong! Depression usually is an integral part of the disease in lupus, often improving strikingly when the lupus is treated. Indeed, some lupus patients who flare after pregnancy are labelled as having puerperal depression.

Headache

Another major feature of lupus is headache; any type of headache can occur, ranging from mild to very severe, including 'cluster headache' and migraine. Headache and migraine are strongly associated with the antiphospholipid (Hughes) syndrome, often improving or even disappearing with anticoagulant treatment (see Chapter 23).

Lupus over time

In many patients, as the decades go by, lupus settles down. Indeed more and more patients these days are eventually weaned off all drugs. Despite this optimistic outlook, many patients still suffer many flares of the disease. The unpredictability of lupus is what makes it so difficult to gauge treatment precisely for many patients.

Late complications

Even when the disease has gone quiet (ie, into remission), there are reasons for vigilance. Prolonged steroid treatment can lead to longer term complications, which can be identified and treated early in many cases. These include osteoporosis, bone softening and cataracts. Some lupus patients develop artery complications including heart attacks, and much effort is now focused on prevention, for example by maintaining a healthy diet, controlling cholesterol, avoiding smoking and, in those patients with sticky blood (see Chapter 14), using anti-clotting medicines such as low-dose aspirin.

My children

As has been stated, there is a definite, albeit weak, genetic tendency in lupus. If any patient is worried about their offspring having lupus, then a simple blood test (ANA) is usually adequate to screen for lupus. The most appropriate time to test (especially in girls who are more likely to be affected) is in the teens after puberty.

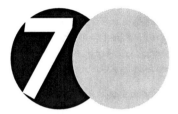

The skin

Introduction

The word 'lupus' (wolf) comes from the old idea that skin lesions on the face resembled wolf bites.

The skin is frequently involved in lupus. Almost any type of skin rash can occur – some of the main skin patterns are described below.

Key points

- 'Butterfly' rash on face
- Rashes on hands and elbows
- Discoid lupus can cause scarring
- Livedo (blotchy circulation) is common
- Plaquenil® is a safe and useful medicine

Systemic lupus erythematosus: skin patterns

The classical picture is of the pinkish, flat rash spread either diffusely or patchily over the face, trunk and limbs. On the face, it can appear in a butterfly rash across the cheeks and nose. It commonly also affects the V of the neck, the tips of the ear lobes and the eyebrows.

The hands and elbows are often involved. On the elbows, there may be small (1 mm) red spots, while on the hands, the picture can vary from severe (a peeling red rash especially on the palms) to mild (pinkish/red discoloration at the nail beds). Although the skin rash is characteristically made worse by sunlight exposure (eg, after a summer vacation), this is not always the case.

Hair loss is a common association, sometimes widespread and severe (eg, hair on the pillow in the morning, not simply on the comb). In systemic lupus, the hair generally grows back fully with successful treatment.

Subacute cutaneous lupus erythematosus (SCLE)

This is a very characteristic skin rash that once seen is never forgotten. The lesions are usually circular or geographic with a distinct border. They often occur on the chest and upper arm.

This rash is associated with a specific blood antibody called anti-Ro (see Chapter 14). It is very sensitive to UV light, and fortunately usually responds very well to antimalarial treatment. It usually has a good prognosis. The circular nature of the skin lesions means that sometimes the condition is mistaken for a fungal infection.

In pregnancy, anti-Ro antibodies can cross the placenta, and occasionally, babies born to anti-Ro-positive mothers develop a very similar rash, which disappears as the weeks go by and the mother's anti-Ro antibodies are cleared away.

Discoid lupus

This is predominantly a skin condition, with only 5% or so of patients developing systemic lupus. Nevertheless, it can be a serious and debilitating condition. The skin becomes roughened and scaly as well as inflamed, and the continuing process can lead to permanent scarring. Unfortunately the main lesions are often on the face and cheeks, nose, ears and scalp, where severe hair loss can occur. Mouth ulcers can be an unpleasant feature. Patchy lesions (sometimes looking like psoriasis) can occur on the arms, legs, abdomen, and hands. The nails can become affected with thickening, ridging and damage.

In general, discoid lupus has a completely different appearance from the rashes of systemic lupus. While discoid skin lesions can be severe, the majority do respond to treatment (generally initially with antimalarial drugs).

There is a 5% risk of systemic (internal) disease, and because some patients with discoid lupus also have Hughes syndrome, a full investigation is always advisable.

Livedo

This is the name given to a skin condition in which the skin appears mottled, giving a 'map of the word' appearance. It is always worse in cold weather. Many healthy people get livedo, for example, young women in particular get livedo on the knees. However, prominent and widespread livedo can indicate one of a number of health problems, particularly those affecting the circulation.

There is one condition especially associated with livedo – Hughes syndrome. Patients with sticky blood (including lupus patients with the condition) frequently have livedo, a telltale sign helpful in diagnosis.

The livedo itself does not constitute a major clinical problem. It often improves when anti-clotting treatment is started.

Chilblains

Some patients develop cold finger and toe circulation, leading to small painful sores (chilblains) on the tips of the digits. In some patients, the tendency to chilblains goes back to childhood, antedating the diagnosis of lupus by many years. Some dermatologists give the name lupus pernio to a particularly prominent form of circulation change with chilblains. However, the presence of these lesions, whilst unpleasant, does not confer any different (or worse) outlook for lupus in general.

Lupus profundus

Just to complete the list, lupus profundus is a rare type of lupus that affects the deeper tissues under the skin, notably the fat. The condition is characterised by uncomfortable or even painful areas of lumpiness under the skin, which leads to visible (and sometimes disfiguring) pits and bumps on the arms, legs, trunk, and unfortunately, occasionally on the face. Although it is an unpleasant and occasionally disfiguring condition, it rarely affects internal organs such as the kidney.

Treatment

Treatment of skin lupus is usually very effective. The mainstay of treatment is the antimalarial drug family – Plaquenil® (hydroxychloroquine) is the first and best choice, and Mepacrine® can be used for more resistant cases.

For patients with more severe skin problems, especially for more resistant cases of discoid lupus or lupus profundus, a number of other drugs are used, with varying degrees of success. These drugs include thalidomide (limited to non-childbearing patients), azathioprine, methotrexate, mofetil and, occasionally, intravenous immunoglobulins.

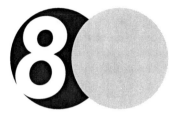

8

The kidney

Introduction

In the old days, lupus was feared mostly for its risk of kidney disease. Kidney failure was widely regarded as one of the natural outcomes of lupus. Fortunately, all that has changed, largely due to earlier diagnosis and effective treatment.

Key points

- Kidney inflammation can be 'silent'
- Blood and urine tests are vital
- Kidney biopsy may be needed
- Can respond fully to treatment

How does the kidney work?

The kidney is the body's filter. It has the amazing ability to sort out the wanted and unwanted components of the blood, getting rid of waste in the urine. The microscopic individual filters in the kidney are called glomeruli, and it is these delicate filters that can become damaged by inflammation in lupus.

The blood flow through the kidney is immense, and the brilliance of the design of the kidney centres on the close proximity of blood capillaries to the filtering apparatus.

It is not surprising that any interruption of blood flow, for example from thrombosis in Hughes syndrome or from inflammation in lupus, can quickly damage this delicate organ. This damage is irreparable unless treatment is started in good time.

Lupus

In lupus, the kidney can be damaged by two processes: blood clotting and inflammation.

Inflammation of the kidney, if unchecked, goes through four stages seen under the microscope on kidney biopsy:

1 The first stage is the invasion of the kidney by inflammation cells, a bit like busy bees around a flower.

2 In the second stage, there is the beginning of damage to the filters (the glomeruli).

3 In the third stage, there is progressive scarring of the glomeruli.

4 In the fourth stage there is more scarring of the glomeruli leading, in extreme cases, to a totally scarred, non-functioning kidney.

Obviously, the aim of treatment is to catch the disease before permanent scarring occurs; the good news is that this can usually be achieved.

Tests

These are described in more detail in Chapter 17. By far the most important is urine testing. This usually gives the earliest indication of kidney inflammation. Blood tests monitor potentially more serious kidney disease, while a kidney biopsy gives the most definitive picture of the state of the disease.

Urine testing

Normal urine is clear, with little or no protein content, no infection and no blood cells.

Increasing amounts of protein in the urine is usually the earliest sign of kidney problems. Small amounts are detected by the well known stick testing (eg, Multistix® or Albustix®). When there is heavy protein loss, a 24 hour urine sample is sometimes ordered, to quantify the loss more precisely.

The sample is sent to the laboratory where it is spun down (centrifuged) and inspected under the microscope for blood cells and bacteria.

Blood tests

The three major blood test indicators are urea, creatinine and albumin. When the glomeruli filters are damaged, toxic waste (including the chemicals urea and creatinine) build up in the bloodstream. By contrast, the level of blood protein (albumin) can fall if there is sufficient loss of protein in the urine. These three measurements are part of the routine investigation in lupus.

Renal biopsy

A fine needle biopsy of the kidney is usually recommended in a patient with clear signs of kidney disease, especially in newly diagnosed patients. The aim of the biopsy is to assess the stage of progress of the disease (eg, whether there is any scarring).

In most centres, biopsy is carried out in the X-ray department under screen guidance. The procedure requires a small injection of local anaesthetic in the loin, and has a remarkably safe record. There is a small chance of bleeding into the urine following biopsy and patients are therefore monitored for 24 hours afterwards.

Treatment

The aims of treatment are twofold: to treat the kidney inflammation itself (usually with a combination of steroids and immunosuppressive drugs), and to treat the parallel and related conditions such as raised blood pressure, raised cholesterol and fluid retention.

Fortunately, total kidney failure in lupus is becoming less and less common, as more effective treatments are being developed that can be used early in the disease.

None the less, for those patients requiring dialysis, lupus itself does not present any major additional problems. For those lupus patients coming to kidney transplantation, the outlook is enormously improved. Indeed one of the unexpected findings of the transplant era is that in lupus patients, the disease itself rarely flares after kidney transplant. Some consolation!

9

Heart and lungs

Introduction

Although the heart and lungs
are separate organs, they are
intimately linked; they are
packed neatly together
within the chest, and interact
functionally together to pump
the oxygen supply around the
body.

Key points

- 1 in 1,000 babies have a slow
  pulse (heart block)

- Heart murmurs occur in some
  patients

- 'Sticky blood' can cause lung
  clots

- Pericarditis and pleurisy respond
  to treatment

Structure of the heart

The heart is a muscular pump. It has three main layers:
an outer sausage skin (the pericardium), the muscle
layer (the myocardium) and the inside lining, including the valves
(the endocardium). All three layers can be attacked by lupus.

An active muscular organ such as the heart depends critically on
a good blood supply. This is provided by the coronary arteries.
It is here that things can go dramatically awry: the three main

branches of the coronary artery can become blocked or cut off. This can give rise to chest pain (ie, angina) or, worse, a more severe blockage leading to a heart attack (ie, a lack of oxygen to a portion of the heart muscle).

Coronary artery disease and heart attacks are among the epidemics of western society and lupus patients, unfortunately, are particularly at risk.

Pericarditis

Inflammation of the surrounding of the heart (pericarditis) is a common feature of lupus, particularly in the early acute stage or in a flare-up.

The classical symptom is chest pain – often sharp and situated in the centre of the chest. Sometimes it is worse in certain positions. The pain is usually different from the crushing pain of angina, but not always so.

Associated with the chest pain is shortness of breath. When the double sausage skin of the pericardium is inflamed, the usual smooth surfaces become roughened and rub together. Often, doctors can hear this rub through the stethoscope as a characteristic scratching noise with each heart beat. The inflammation then creates fluid (as it does in the skin with a blister) and this fluid can accumulate between the two layers of the pericardium – this is known as a pericardial effusion. In extreme cases, this fluid accumulation can impair the heart beat and lead to extreme distress, shortness of breath, and pump failure with accumulation of fluid throughout the body.

Heart muscle

Fortunately, a direct attack on the heart muscle in lupus is unusual. A more common, and an important problem, is coronary artery thrombosis and furring (atheroma).

Now that survival in lupus is hugely improved, with patients leading full lives and having normal life spans, a new problem has been recognised. A second disease peak has been picked up in lupus patients in their 40s and 50s – blood vessel problems, notably heart attack and stroke.

The cause of this increased propensity to atheroma and heart attack in some patients is now the focus of intensive study, but the solution remains elusive. The usual suspects include prolonged steroid use, kidney disease and raised blood pressure, but in reality none of these fully explains the phenomenon.

One suspect is sticky blood due to Hughes syndrome (also called antiphospholipid syndrome). Studies have shown a tendency in some Hughes syndrome patients to develop constrictions, or stenosis, of certain arteries including the coronary arteries. Logically therefore, the appropriate use of low dose aspirin (as well as good control of cholesterol) may reduce the risk of later artery clots and heart attacks.

The valves

It has been known for many decades that the heart valves can be affected in a small number of patients with lupus. Indeed, the unusual condition of heart valve thickening with blood clots on their surfaces is widely known as Libman–Sacks endocarditis. Recently, however, with the discovery of the antiphospholipid syndrome, it appears likely that valve problems in lupus are more closely linked to this condition.

The main symptom of heart valve involvement is shortness of breath. The 'whooshing' noise made by a leaky heart valve can usually be heard through a stethoscope, though more detailed heart tests are needed to determine the size of the leak.

Benign murmurs, requiring no specific therapy, are common – not only in lupus but also in the population at large. Severe valve disease requiring surgery is rare.

Congenital heart block

A rare heart defect, congenital heart block, has been noted in 1 in 1,000 infants born of lupus (and Sjögren's syndrome) mothers. This defect in the heart's conduction tissue results in a slow pulse rate (around 40 per minute) in the offspring. It is a serious manifestation and more often than not requires the insertion of a pacemaker into the young infant's heart.

The condition is limited to children of mothers carrying the antibody called anti-Ro and is thought to be due to the mother's antibody crossing the placenta and reacting with the fetus' heart conduction tissue.

Pleurisy

One of the most common manifestations of active lupus is pleurisy which is due to inflammation of the lining of the lungs. Like the heart, the lungs are surrounded by two thin 'sausage skin' layers called the pleura. These normally move together painlessly during breathing. When the pleura become inflamed, they become roughened, stick together, and cause pain on inspiration (breathing in). This rubbing together can sometimes be heard as a pleural rub through the stethoscope.

Lung clots

One of the serious complications of a blood clot (eg, a deep vein thrombosis in the leg or pelvis) is a pulmonary embolus, that is, a broken-off piece of clot travelling to the lung. This is usually a dramatic and life threatening event, associated with chest pain and collapse. However, in some cases (notably again in those patients with Hughes syndrome and its clotting tendency), the lung clots may go relatively unnoticed. An untreated build up of lung clots over a period of months and years is one of the causes of the serious medical condition known as pulmonary hypertension.

Pulmonary hypertension

Hypertension means raised blood pressure. In pulmonary hypertension the pressure is on the right side of the heart, the side which pumps blood around the lungs. The main clinical effect of pressure build-up is shortness of breath. This serious condition, measured by a series of cardiology tests, was once considered untreatable. Now, however, there is more optimism with a group of exciting new medications coming on stream.

Pulmonary fibrosis

Another cause of shortness of breath, though completely distinct from the clotting conditions described above, is pulmonary fibrosis.

In this condition, the normally soft, delicate lung tissue becomes scarred. I liken it to the effect you get when you lick freshly spun candy floss – the edges become stuck together and less mobile.

Pulmonary fibrosis has many causes, and is seen as an unusual complication in a number of diseases including rheumatoid arthritis. It is, in fact, very unusual in lupus.

Infection

No account of the lung in lupus would be complete without mentioning infection of the chest. Individuals with impaired immune defences or those on strong immunosuppressive drugs are more prone to infection. These infections include tuberculosis, an infection once again on the increase. In any patient with unexplained recurrent cough or chest problems, the doctor should be on the alert for a lurking infection.

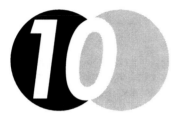

The brain

Introduction

The brain is a miracle machine. And yet in some ways, it is remarkably stupid. If interfered with (eg, poor blood supply or inflammation) it has fairly limited ways of complaining – headaches, memory loss, depression, strokes, seizures – features which are shared with a whole host of other conditions.

Key points

- Brain involvement in lupus takes many forms

- Symptoms include: migraine, depression, memory loss, seizures

- Brain problems often due to 'sticky blood'

- Can be treated successfully

And yet the problems (as well as possible solutions) can be looked at in a fairly simple way. In lupus there are two main threats to organs such as the brain: inflammation (direct attack by lupus) and poor circulation (sludging or stickiness of the blood in patients with antiphospholipid antibodies and Hughes syndrome). Clearly, different treatments are needed in the two situations – steroids and anti-inflammatory medicines in the first, and anti-clotting agents (eg, aspirin, warfarin, etc.) in the second. Arguably the biggest advance in lupus in recent years has come from the observation that much of the brain problem in lupus comes from sticky blood, which is potentially very treatable.

The outlook or prognosis for brain disease, provided that the danger of blood clotting is recognised and dealt with, is surprisingly good. I have many patients who have had a distressing past history of depression, memory problems, fits, phobias and even psychosis, who are now leading completely normal lives, free of neuro-psychiatric symptoms.

Anatomy

Medical students learn about the central nervous system, comprising the brain and spinal cord (the computer), and the peripheral nervous system (the wiring to the far flung areas) from the scalp to the toes, and doctors are trained to distinguish between these vitally different areas. However, all families who have looked after relativeswith stroke, for instance, know the broad outline of brain problems which will depend on the site of the damage. For example, speech problems or a stroke indicate one-sided weakness, balance problems (the cerebellum), leg weakness and bladder disturbance (the spinal cord), and so on. Signs pointing to peripheral nervous system problems include numbness, pins and needles, formication (an odd name derived from ants where there is a feeling of crawling sensations under the skin), and the finding by the doctor of absent (or impaired) reflexes with the tendon hammer.

Obviously, it is the highly complex brain which gives rise to the huge variety of features, ranging from absences, to panic attacks, depression, and memory problems.

Migraine and headache

Headache has long been considered a common problem in lupus. A big breakthrough came with the discovery of antiphospholipid syndrome.We now recognise that by far the most important cause of headaches in lupus patients is sticky blood. Many lupus patients have a history of teenage migraine, often going away for years before returning. It is absolutely critical to

'Did you suffer from childhood, or teenage, headache or migraine?'

'Yes doctor, I missed days from school, a big problem.'

test for Hughes syndrome (aPL testing – see Chapter 16). One of the most satisfying results in lupus is the improvement and even disappearance of headache (and memory problems) when anti-clotting medicine is started.

Stroke and transient ischaemic attack (TIA)

The most feared complication of lupus is stroke or, its early warning cousin, TIA. The latter is a related but less severe event involving a period of difficulty in speech or movement lasting from seconds to minutes.

We now recognise that, in lupus, stroke (like headache and many of the other conditions discussed in this chapter) is the extreme consequence of clotting due to Hughes syndrome. Early treatment is vital and effective. A patient found to be positive for antiphospholipid antibodies (aCL and LA positive – see Chapter 16) and especially with small 'dots' on the brain MRI scan should be treated urgently with anticoagulants such as heparin or warfarin. If treatment is fast and effective, the patient is spared any worsening of what could be a clotting disaster.

Depression

Depression, in all its forms, is an important part of lupus and is often under-recognised. Too often, mild depression is attributed simply to the stress of having a chronic illness (eg, fatigue, joint pains). But in many cases, the depression can dramatically improve if the underlying lupus is recognised and treated successfully. Often it is difficult for doctors and patients alike to dissect out a depression component from all the other features of the disease. The decision of whether to add anti-depressant to the overall lupus treatment is a difficult one and requires experience on the doctor's part.

Psychosis

Very rarely, the brain involvement in lupus leads to more severe brain disturbance, including psychosis. During such an episode the patient may hear voices. The good news is that even in the most severe examples (eg, when the patient has been thought to have schizophrenia), the outcome is usually good. With treatment (usually both lupus treatment and anti-psychotic medication) there is every reason to expect full recovery.

Memory loss

This is a major feature of patients with Hughes syndrome (sticky blood). Given that the brain needs a good circulation to function, it is not surprising that impairment of the oxygen supply leads to a variety of symptoms. Memory loss varies from mild ('I have to write everything down') to severe and more frightening (eg, one patient could not remember which exit of the traffic roundabout led to her home). One of the truly dramatic advances in lupus has been the memory improvement in patients with lupus and Hughes syndrome when treated with anti-clotting agents such as aspirin, heparin or warfarin.

Balance and hearing

We now recognise that many of the neurological features of lupus (eg, balance problems, seizures and atypical multiple sclerosis) are closely linked to antiphospholipid syndrome (Hughes syndrome) and may well respond better to anti-clotting medicines than to steroids.

Balance problems are usually due to circulation impairment in the middle ear. Not surprisingly, ringing in the ears (tinnitus) is sometimes a feature.

Vision disturbances

Vision problems range from focusing difficulty to loss of vision. There are many causes: for example, drugs such as steroids can affect the pressure in the eye and alter focal length. Alterations in blood pressure and circulation to the eye can also lead to a variety of symptoms. One of the most dramatic (and potentially treatable) symptoms is sudden loss of part or all of the field of vision, secondary to blood clotting in Hughes syndrome.

Multiple sclerosis

A number of our patients with lupus and Hughes syndrome who have features such as balance disorder, pins and needles, and visual disturbance are, not surprisingly, labelled as having possible multiple sclerosis (MS).

Distinguishing the two conditions can be very difficult but vitally important, and it is one of the main clinical research projects in our unit.

St. Vitus' dance

Medically known as chorea, this jerking movement of the head, arms and body, is one of a variety of movement disorders seen in lupus and Hughes syndrome. Neurologists recognise a wide spectrum, ranging from periodic 'tics' through to cases resembling Parkinson's disease.

Seizures

Occasionally lupus is characterised by the dramatic development of fits or seizures. Again, it is now recognised that this brain disturbance is often associated with sticky blood and can respond to anti-clotting drugs. This observation is having a profound effect on the subject of neurology in general. For example, one recent study suggested that up to 20% of all cases of unexpected teenage epilepsy tested positive for antiphospholipid antibodies!

Undiagnosed lupus

From the above, it is obvious that brain involvement in lupus and Hughes syndrome takes many forms. There are, without doubt, a number of patients out there with memory loss, or seizures, or the symptoms of MS, for example, in whom lupus or Hughes syndrome is the underlying cause. So treatable! So important!

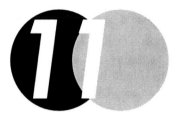

The blood

Introduction

Blood is composed of a liquid plasma, in which there are three floating components – red cells, white cells and platelets.

In lupus, levels of any or all of these three components can be reduced.

Key points

- Red and white cell counts are often low; platelets may be low too

- Anaemia may also be due to bleeding

- All three components of the blood may be affected but respond well to treatment

Red cells

These cells carry haemoglobin, which is vital for carrying oxygen around the blood; a low level of red blood cells (and therefore low haemoglobin) is called anaemia. In practical terms, there are two main causes of anaemia in lupus: blood loss (iron-deficiency anaemia) and haemolysis (damage of red blood cells).

The two most common causes of iron-deficiency anaemia in lupus are (in women) heavy periods, and blood loss from the digestive tract (often due to irritation by medicines, notably the anti-inflammatory drugs used for arthritis).

The signs and symptoms of anaemia are fatigue, breathlessness and pallor of the skin. Confirmation of the iron-deficiency diagnosis is usually made by measurement of serum iron levels. Obviously, if blood loss from the stomach or intestine is suspected, further investigation such as gastroscopy may be required.

A less common, though important, cause of anaemia in lupus is haemolytic anaemia. Antibodies directed against red blood cells make them more fragile. Anaemia (which can be sudden and severe) results from the spontaneous breakdown of the red blood cells in the circulation.

White cells

The white blood cells form a vital defence mechanism. The two main types of white cells are lymphocytes (the immune cells) and polymorphs (also called neutrophils), which are the cells responsible for catching and ingesting bacteria.

In lupus, it is almost the rule that the white blood count is on the low side (eg, $3,000\ 10^9/L$). In most cases this slightly low count appears to cause no clinical problems. Occasionally, however, the total count falls severely, leaving the patient at an increased risk for infections.

Platelets

Platelets are minute sausage-like particles that play a vital role in blood clotting. In the normal blood stream they flow freely, but following any damage, such as a cut, they clump together to form part of a blood clot to stop the loss of blood. In lupus, and especially in Hughes syndrome, the antibodies can affect and damage the platelets. The result can be either a fall in platelet numbers or, alternatively, abnormal sticking together to form spontaneous thrombosis.

Low platelet counts can lead to bruising and bleeding. This condition is known as thrombocytopenia, and when it occurs by itself and with no other evidence of lupus, it is known as idiopathic thrombocytopenic purpura (ITP).

In summary, all three major components of the blood – the white cells, the red cells and the platelets – can be affected in lupus. Fortunately all three deficiencies (cytopenias) generally respond well to treatment.

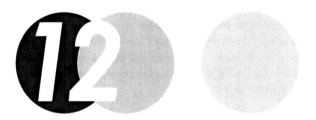

Pregnancy and lupus

Introduction

How things have changed. Forty years ago, and even more recently, lupus was widely regarded as a contraindication to pregnancy. Many thousands

Key points

- Pregnancy is successful in most
- Miscarriage is linked to 'sticky blood'
- Risk of lupus flare after delivery

of lupus patients were advised against pregnancy at all costs. Now, pregnancy in lupus is accepted in most circumstances, though special care is needed. Specialist pregnancy clinics are opening all over the world. However, the success of pregnancy in lupus depends heavily on the lupus being under good or reasonable control.

There are two particular problems for patients who are pregnant with lupus. First, there is a higher risk of miscarriage, and second, there is an increased chance of a flare of lupus after the baby is born.

Management of pregnancy

Ideally, pregnancy care should be shared between obstetricians and lupus doctors. Happily, with the advent of combined lupus pregnancy clinics, this is happening more and more. In most patients, the pregnancy is uneventful and managed in the same way as in women without lupus. The major advance has come from the discovery of the antiphospholipid syndrome and its impact on the prevention of miscarriage.

Miscarriage

The presence of antiphospholipid antibodies (see Chapter 14) is associated, tragically, with an increased risk of pregnancy loss not only early on during the first 12 weeks, but sometimes later in the pregnancy. The most likely cause is clotting of the placenta, leading to a poor blood supply to the fetus. Other mechanisms such as inflammation in the placenta may also be involved. Whatever the mechanism, treatment with anti-clotting drugs (eg, aspirin or heparin) has revolutionised the outcome for these pregnancies. There is still debate about the relative merits of aspirin and heparin. However, in those aPL positive women with previous pregnancy loss or previous thrombosis, more and more doctors are turning to low molecular weight heparin. While this means daily self-injection for most of the nine months, the outcome is worth the inconvenience.

Long term heparin has been linked to the development of osteoporosis in some patients, though with the newer, low molecular weight products (eg, Fragmin®, Clexane®) this seems to be extremely unusual.

Another advance in lupus pregnancy monitoring has come with the scanning technique known as 'Doppler'. This scan, which shows the pulse blood supply to the fetus, acts as an important early warning alarm in later pregnancy. A falling Doppler blood flow to the intra-uterine infant is usually an indication for early caesarean section before fetal distress can set in.

Puerperium

Pregnancy does not normally affect the frequency of flares. However, once the baby is born, there is an increased chance of a flare of lupus. It is important, therefore, that patients are monitored more closely during the first few months after childbirth, so that an increase in treatment can be given where appropriate.

Breast feeding is certainly allowed in most patients, and, perhaps surprisingly, most of the major drugs used in lupus are allowed during breast feeding.

The baby

The offspring of most lupus patients are healthy and there is no need to test for lupus. The two rare complications of neonatal skin rash and congenital heart block (slow pulse) are confined to mothers with anti-Ro antibodies (see Chapter 9).

Infertility

Some patients, mainly those with active disease and some women with anti-phosopholipid antibodies (aPL), experience difficulties in becoming pregnant. In the case of the former, it is advisable for the disease to be brought under better control, with steroids if necessary. In aPL positive women, aspirin is usually tried on the theoretical basis that blood supply to the early embryo is improved. Others advocate heparin, and many IVF clinics now add heparin to their standard IVF cocktail. Overall, the fertility rate in lupus is the same as in the overall female population. Secondly, lupus is not a contraindication to IVF in those women needing this treatment.

Drugs

Many of the drugs used in lupus, for instance Plaquenil® and steroids, are safe both in pregnancy and during breast feeding, but others, notably some of the immunosuppressive drugs, are not. In general patients on strong immunosuppressive drugs, such as methotrexate, mofetil and cyclophosphamide, stop this treatment six months before embarking on a pregnancy.

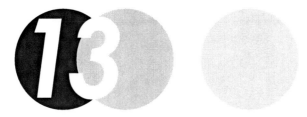

Sjögren's syndrome

Introduction

Many diseases are named after the physicians who first described the condition. Some are rare – 'small print' conditions – others are common and important, both in terms of frequency, but also in their contribution to medical knowledge in its broader sense. One disease falling into the second group is Sjögren's syndrome.

Key points

- Symptoms include: 'scratchy' eyes, dry mouth

- Associated with Hughes syndrome and hypothyroidism

- Under-recognised and under-treated condition

- Outlook is good following correct diagnosis

Background

Henrick Sjögren, a Swedish eye doctor, described a triad of dry eyes, dry mouth, and aches and pains. We now know that Sjögren's is an autoimmune condition – a cousin of lupus – usually presenting in slightly older individuals (eg, 30–60) than the average lupus age group. Although potentially less life threatening than lupus,

Sjögren's can cause chronic medical problems, often because it remains undiagnosed and untreated.

Clinical features

The main features are usually less dramatic than in lupus and hence often go undiagnosed.

Fatigue, as in lupus, is common. Often unhelpfully labelled as fibromyalgia or ME, it is the main feature of Sjögren's.

Allergies are common and these can include food allergies (often important and very real in Sjögren's), skin allergies and general allergies. One dramatic feature is Septrin® allergy. Septrin®, a sulphonamide-like antibiotic, once very fashionable for the treatment of cystitis, almost universally causes allergy (sometimes severe) in Sjögren's patients. It is so common as to be, in my opinion, almost a diagnostic feature of the syndrome. Aches and pains are common, as is gland swelling. A number of patients with Sjögren's give a past history of severe glandular fever in their teens. Indeed the EB virus, the cause of glandular fever, has long been implicated as a cause of Sjögren's.

Joints

Aches and pains are common, and can affect muscles and tendons as well as joints. Sometimes the joints can become quite severely swollen, resembling rheumatoid arthritis. Fortunately, in the majority of cases, this pattern does not progress to chronic, disabling rheumatoid disease.

Eyes

Many patients do not realise they have dry eyes, but they may notice a scratching of the eyes, a stickiness of the eyes on waking, or light sensitivity and the need for sunglasses. A very important test known as Schirmer's test, is used in the diagnosis. This consists of hooking a standard strip of blotting paper over the lower eyelid for 5 minutes. Normally this irritation provokes enough eye watering to soak the paper, but in Sjögren's it remains dry.

Other 'dry' organs

The dryness associated with Sjögren's is caused by an infiltration of the mucus glands by immune cells. As well as the lachrymal glands of the eyes, the salivary glands can also be affected (leading to dry mouth and a risk of dental caries). The dryness can affect other mucus membranes, leading to difficulty in swallowing, a dry cough, vaginal dryness (resulting in painful intercourse and risk of vaginal thrush) and even dryness of the bladder and urethra leading to recurrent (but non-infectious) cystitis.

Associated illness

There are two major autoimmune associations of Sjögren's – Hughes syndrome and hypothyroidism (underactive thyroid). A significant proportion of Sjögren's patients (between 10–40%) have Hughes syndrome (sticky blood). This commonly leads to headaches, memory loss, balance problems and other features of Hughes syndrome. As these symptoms usually respond to anti-clotting treatment such as aspirin, it is important for doctors to pick up on the link between Hughes syndrome and Sjögren's syndrome.

A second common association is low thyroid, another autoimmune condition. Autoimmune hypothyroidism (also called Hashimoto's disease) can lead to fatigue and sluggishness, feeling the cold, and mental slowness which means it can be easy for doctor's to miss, especially in the context of Sjögren's syndrome, and yet it is very treatable.

A third associated condition, though much rarer, is non-Hodgkin's lymphoma (NHL). This malignancy of the lymphatic system, now usually very treatable, is seen more frequently not only in patients with autoimmune diseases such as Sjögren's, but also in their relatives. Earlier reports tended to over estimate the frequency of NHL in Sjögren's, concentrating on patients with Sjögren's with major gland swelling, rather than those patients presenting with a more typical clinical picture.

This complication is rare but should of course be considered if prominent gland swelling becomes a feature.

Treatment

The general symptoms of Sjögren's usually respond to quinine, given in the form of hydroxychloroquine (Plaquenil®) 1–2 doses daily, although some cases will respond over time to a lower dose, such as 3 tablets a week. Plaquenil® is a safe and mild medicine, and it has a marvellous beneficial effect in many Sjögren's patients. Aspirin is the main first-line choice for the features of Hughes syndrome.

For the dry eyes, 'artificial tears' (eg, hypromellose, a bland cellulose like lubricant) are used. Dry mouth is more difficult; most patients resort to frequent sips of water or the occasional use of sugarless chewing gum. For some patients with major dry mouth problems, a medicine called Salagen® (pilocarpine) is occasionally used.

Prognosis

The outlook for patients with Sjögren's, given a correct diagnosis and treatment, is good. Contrary to some opinions, it does not develop into lupus. Having said this, it is still a hugely under-recognised and under-treated condition.

Hughes syndrome (antiphospholipid syndrome)

Introduction

Often called sticky blood syndrome, this condition, in which the blood has a tendency to sludge or clot, was first described in detail a mere 25 years ago in 1983.

It is another cousin of lupus (ie, it is an autoimmune disease).

Key points

- Also called 'sticky blood syndrome'
- Headache and migraine are common
- Test blood for anti-phospholipid antibodies
- Treat with anticoagulants
- Risk of miscarriage if untreated

In this case, the offending antibodies disrupt the membranes of the platelets and blood vessels resulting in thrombosis. These vital membranes consist of complex molecules such as phospholipids, and the title given to the syndrome was the antiphospholipid syndrome (APS). Such has been the explosion of knowledge of this syndrome that international conferences on APS are now held every second year. In 1992, I was honoured that my colleagues recognised my discovery of the condition with the eponym Hughes syndrome.

Main features

Under normal conditions, blood does not clot. The blood cells and platelets flow cleanly along the veins and arteries like trout in a stream. In Hughes syndrome sudden (or gradual, more subtle) clotting can occur, leading, for example, to thrombosis (clot) in an arm or leg, which is known as deep vein thrombosis (DVT).

This tendency to clotting can affect any part of the body, including delicate organs such as the brain. Many patients carrying antiphospholipid antibodies (aPL) are asymptomatic, the thrombosis only happening when other known risk factors are present (eg, after a long haul flight, starting the oral contraceptive pill, pregnancy). The two, seemingly, most susceptible organs are the brain and, in pregnancy, the placenta.

Brain

Just as a car engine stutters when deprived of the correct mix of gasoline, so does the brain with sticky blood. Almost every neurological feature has been reported in Hughes syndrome, including fits, balance problems, visual disturbance (some Hughes syndrome patients are wrongly diagnosed with multiple sclerosis) and movement disorders. However, the two most prominent symptoms are headache and poor memory.

Headaches can start as early as childhood, and are often migrainous with nausea and flashing lights. There is often a family history of migraine.

Memory loss varies from mild ('I couldn't find the right words') to severe (ie, so much so that the patient often fears Alzheimer's disease).

The most feared complication is stroke; it has been estimated that up to 1 in 5 of all strokes in people under 45 are due to Hughes syndrome. The good news is that these can be prevented.

Skin and other organs

Poor circulation in the skin leads to a mottled (corned beef skin) appearance called livedo reticularis.

In the heart, poor circulation can lead to chest pain (angina), in the lungs to shortness of breath, in the kidney to raised blood pressure and in the stomach to abdominal pain after meals. In the blood the platelet numbers can be reduced (thrombocytopenia).

Occasionally, clotting can become widespread and acute, leading to a life threatening, very rare condition dubbed the catastrophic antiphospholipid syndrome.

Pregnancy

Clotting in the placenta can lead to impaired blood supply to the fetus, leading to miscarriage (or even late pregnancy loss). Indeed Hughes syndrome has been called the most common *treatable* cause of recurrent pregnancy loss. Some women suffer six, eight, ten or even more miscarriages.

The diagnosis and treatment (with either aspirin or heparin) of Hughes syndrome has proved to be one of the success stories of modern medicine, with the successful pregnancy rate rising from 18% in 1985 to over 90% in most modern lupus pregnancy clinics.

Infertility

In some women, recurrent very early pregnancy loss leads to a label of infertility. Indeed, many infertility clinics now routinely test for aPL, and some include heparin, for example, in their treatment protocol. However, the degree of contribution of aPL to overall infertility figures is unclear at the present time.

Diagnosis

☑ Anticardiolipin antibodies

☑ Lupus anticoagulant

Diagnosis is confirmed by two relatively simple blood tests, now carried out in laboratories throughout the world.

These blood tests have rather complicated (and confusing) names. The reason for needing to tick the box for two rather than one test is that a number of patients with Hughes syndrome are only positive for one or the other.

Treatment

Currently, there are three main choices: aspirin (75–100 mg daily or clopidogrel [Plavix®] for those intolerant of aspirin), heparin, and warfarin.

Aspirin is satisfactory for most milder cases, while warfarin is necessary for those with clear cut thrombosis, or with more brain involvement. Heparin can only be given by injection. It is used as a first-line immediate treatment for thrombosis, and also if warfarin needs to be stopped (eg, prior to and during an operation).

In pregnancy, warfarin is contraindicated especially, during the first half of pregnancy. Daily heparin injections are used when there has been thrombosis or in patients with a number of previous miscarriages.

The future

Recognition of the syndrome and its successful treatment have had a major impact in medicine. Up to 1 in 5 of all strokes in people under 45 years old, 1 in 5 recurrent miscarriages, and 1 in 5 DVTs are associated with aPL, not to mention an unknown number of individuals with migraine, multiple sclerosis, memory loss and epilepsy, in whom recognition and treatment of the correct diagnosis could be life altering.

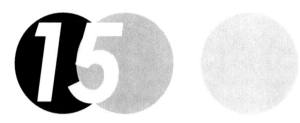

Mixed connective tissue disease (Sharpe's syndrome)

Introduction

All those who treat lupus and related diseases know that, in practice, there is a spectrum of diseases with overlaps, for example, between some cases of rheumatoid arthritis and lupus.

Some of these lupus variants, such as primary Sjögren's syndrome, or Hughes syndrome, however, have a sufficiently distinctive pattern to warrant separate consideration.

Key points

- Symptoms include: Raynaud's (cold hands), joint and muscle pain
- Test for anti-RNP antibodies
- Treatment involves steroids, and steroid-sparing drugs
- Rarely life-threatening, unlikely to progress to lupus or scleroderma
- Serious kidney disease is rare

One such condition is mixed connective tissue disease (Sharpe's syndrome). Although the condition is sometimes derided as being a vague entity, large lupus clinics recognise it as an important and distinct syndrome.

Background

Gordon Sharpe, in the 1960s, recognised a group of patients with a triad of joint pains, muscle pains and Raynaud's phenomenon. These patients were distinct from classical lupus in rarely going on to develop renal disease or the other severe Raynaud's disorder, scleroderma.

They were also distinguished by a blood test, anti-RNP, which is distinct from anti-DNA and other anti-nuclear antibodies.

Joints and muscles

Widespread aches and pains are common. The fingers characteristically develop spindle-shaped swelling. Frequently, the degree of inflammation in the joints, especially the knuckles and fingers, is greater than that seen in lupus, nearer in appearance to rheumatoid arthritis, but usually without the joint damage seen in that disease.

Muscles

Aching muscles are a major feature of mixed connective tissue disorder. Sometimes this spills over into a full picture of muscle inflammation with tenderness, muscle weakness, and abnormal blood tests (raised blood levels of the muscle enzyme CK (creatine kinase).

Raynaud's

In this condition, the fingers (and often the toes) have a tendency to go white, especially in the cold. Classically there are three changes of colour – white, blue, and as the circulation returns, red.

Raynaud's phenomenon is seen in many conditions but with varying intensity. In sclerodoma, it is often severe, while in lupus it is milder. In mixed connective tissue disorder, Raynaud's is prominent and sometimes the most dominant and severe feature of the syndrome.

Other features

As in lupus, inflammation in the lining of the lungs and heart (pleurisy and pericarditis) can occur. Unlike lupus, however, kidney inflammation is rare. Some skin tightness can occur, though progression to scleroderma is very unusual.

Blood tests

The blood test most useful in diagnosis is an antibody test, namely anti-RNP (anti-ribonucleoprotein). This is often present in high concentrations. As RNP is part of the nucleus, the screening ANA (anti-nuclear antibody) is usually positive, sometimes reported by the laboratory as having a speckled pattern. Critically, the specific test for lupus (anti-DNA) is usually negative.

Treatment

Mixed connective tissue disorder, while not usually a life-threatening disease, is often a grumbling and troublesome condition. Steroids are frequently needed, especially if there is muscle inflammation or pleurisy. Steroid-sparing drugs are frequently used, including Plaquenil®, azathioprine, and methotrexate, which is useful if arthritis or muscle inflammation is prominent.

Unfortunately, for patients with Raynaud's, there is no easy answer and although a wide variety of medicines have been used (including Prozac® and Viagra®), none is especially effective. It is hoped that the newer 'magic bullet' monoclonal agents such as rituximab may be more effective.

Prognosis

Mixed connective tissue disorder is a very grumbling condition, but it is rarely life-threatening. Although it shares many features with lupus and scleroderma, it rarely progresses to these diseases.

Antibody tests

LE cell test

In 1948, a big step forward was made in the diagnosis of lupus with the discovery of the LE cell. This was an unusual blood cell which, under the microscope, appeared as a scavenger cell which seemed to have ingested the nucleus of another cell. It was recognised by researchers at the Mayo Clinic, USA, as being relatively specific for lupus, and its detection soon became the standard diagnostic test for lupus.

Unfortunately, the test is cumbersome and lacks accuracy, and has now been largely replaced by more reliable tests such as ANA (anti-nuclear antibody) and Anti-DNA (anti-DNA antibody).

Key points

- ANA – standard screening test, but not highly specific

- DNA – high specific test for lupus

- Anticardiolipin antibodies – test for Hughes syndrome

Anti-nuclear antibody (ANA)

This is now the standard screening test for lupus throughout the world. It is simple to perform in the laboratory and requires only a drop of blood.

Essentially, the patient's serum is placed on a glass slide containing cells (a small sample of tissue). Any anti-nuclear antibodies present in the patient's serum will stick to the nuclei of the cells and are then detected using a fluorescent dye which is visible under a special microscope.

It is common practice to test increasingly dilute samples, thus giving a reading of, for example 1 in 10, 1 in 20, and so on, up to a very strong positive of, say 1 in 1,280. Weak positive results (eg, 1 in 20) are relatively meaningless but a strong positive suggests either lupus or another of the autoimmune diseases.

Although useful as a test, ANA screening is not specific, with positive results also found, for example, in other conditions such as rheumatoid arthritis, Sjögren's syndrome, scleroderma, and with certain medications.

Nevertheless, a positive result should lead on to the very specific test for lupus, the anti-DNA test.

Anti-DNA antibody (Anti-DNA)

In the late 1960s, intense research work was done on the nature of anti-nuclear antibodies. It was soon recognised that of the many reactions with the nucleus, reactivity against DNA was the specific test for lupus.

Over the past four decades, anti-DNA antibody testing has become one of the most specific tests in diagnosing lupus, with a strongly positive test making lupus the most likely diagnosis. False positives in other conditions are extremely rare.

There are a number of ways of measuring anti-DNA antibodies and the results may vary between different laboratories.

As with ANA tests, the result is usually given as a dilution ('titre') with high results being almost conclusive for lupus.

Extractable nuclear antigens (ENA)

The ANAs are in fact reacting against a mixture of chemicals in the cell – DNA, RNA (ribonucleic acid), nucleoproteins and so on. In the early days of ANA research, this mixture was called 'extractable nuclear antigens'. Bit by bit these extracts were identified and given names such as anti-Sm, anti-Ro, anti-La and anti-RNP and so on. Some of these arbitrary titles were named after patients, for example, anti-Sm was first detected in a patient named Smith!

One or two of these antibodies have become very useful diagnostic tools, and are summarised below:

Anti-Sm: Found in lupus.
Of some (limited) value as a back up to anti-DNA.

Anti-Ro: Found in skin lupus. Also in Sjögren's.
Associated with sun-sensitivity, and with the rare problem of cogenital heart block (see Chapter 9).

Anti-La: Similar to anti-Ro.

Anti-RNP: Associated with Raynaud's phenomenon and mixed connective tissue disease (see Chapter 15).

Anti-Jo1: Very specific for a form of muscle disease (myositis).

Anti-Scl70: Found in a number of cases of scleroderma.

Anticardiolipin

The family of antibodies against phospholipids (constituents of platelet and cell membranes) are important markers for the blood clotting disease known as the antiphospholipid syndrome (APS) or Hughes syndrome.

Other antibodies

Over 100 antigen–antibody reactions have now been described. Many of these are seen in lupus patients, but as yet have not achieved a useful role in lupus clinical practice.

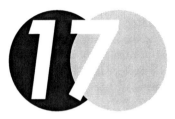

Other tests

Full blood count

All three main components of the blood – the red cells, the white cells and the platelets – can be low in active lupus.

The red cells carry haemoglobin, which is a protein that transports oxygen, and as in any disease, the haemoglobin level can fall (anaemia). The main causes of anaemia in lupus are:

Key points

- ESR – guide to inflammation
- CRP – low in lupus, high in infection
- CPK – test for muscle inflammation
- Urine testing is vital

1 active disease

2 blood loss (eg, heavy periods, indigestion for example brought on by anti-rheumatic drugs)

3 haemolytic anaemia, which is a much rarer cause where the red cells are damaged by antibodies.

The normal white cell count is between 4,000 and 10,000 10^9/L. A raised white count can be a sign of infection, and is also frequently seen in patients on steroids.

More common in lupus is a low white cell count, often between 2,000 and 4,000. Fortunately this order of reduction is usually harmless and it is not uncommon for lupus patients to run low counts year in year out. Finally, in patients on immunosuppressive drugs, it is very important to monitor the blood count as all components of the blood, especially the white count, can fall.

The normal platelet count is over 150,000 10^9/L. Occasionally the platelet count can fall in lupus, especially in those patients with antiphospholipid antibodies. Severe drops in the platelet count (eg, 20,000 or below) are unusual but do occur, and generally require more aggressive therapy, for example a higher dose of steroids.

Erythrocyte sedimentation rate (ESR)

This time-honoured test is used as a barometer of disease activity. Traditionally a sample of blood is sucked up into a calibrated tube (very much like a barometer) and left to stand for one hour. The amount of sedimentation of the red cells is then recorded (under 20 mm being 'within normal', over 100 mm being 'very active'). The test is not specific for lupus, but it does provide a useful guide to progress, especially in patients with rheumatic symptoms.

C-reactive protein (CRP)

This is another test which has been around for a long time, but has found a new use in lupus. In 1980, working with Professor Mark Pepys at Hammersmith Hospital, London, we reported that the level of CRP, while raised in most inflammatory conditions (like ESR), often remained low in lupus patients. Indeed, we even published a paper which suggested that a high ESR/low CRP ratio could be a diagnostic pointer towards lupus. In a lupus patient with infection, however, the CRP did rise. Thus in a sick lupus patient with fever (the 'friday night case') a low CRP suggests lupus, a high CRP suggests infection.

Biochemistry

Routine blood tests for kidney disease include creatinine and urea (levels of which rise when the kidney fails to filter properly) and serum albumin (which falls when the kidney leaks protein into the urine). Tests for liver function include gamma-GT, alkaline phosphatase and alanine transferase (ALT) together with bilirubin. However, direct liver inflammation in lupus is unusual.

Other tests usually included in an automated blood health screen are calcium, phosphate, uric acid (high in cases of gout) and serum iron.

Creatine phosphokinase (CPK)

CPK (also called CK, creatine kinase) is a blood enzyme and a useful marker for muscle inflammation. The normal value of under 150 sometimes rises to over 10,000 in patients with severe muscle inflammation (myositis).

CPK levels also rise physiologically after exercise. A rare side effect of the statin drugs (increasingly used for raised cholesterol) is muscle ache, and in this situation a persistently raised CPK level can prove to be a useful diagnostic aid.

Cholesterol

A blood cholesterol and lipid screen is now considered a vital part of lupus screening in view of the increased tendency of lupus patients to develop atheroma and arterial disease (see Chapter 6). The generally accepted normal upper limit of cholesterol is less than 5 mmol/L, though this target is coming down, especially with the increasing use of statins.

Urine tests

Urine tests are vital in the management of lupus. Routine home testing and clinic visit urine testing is carried out by simple blotting paper sticks that change colour if there is protein, or sugar or blood, for example, in the urine. It is my practice to teach all my patients the technique of urine self-testing.

For more exact analysis, a clear specimen of urine is sent to the lab to be analysed under the microscope.

Normal urine, of course, is clear under the microscope. However any problems are shown up by the presence of white blood cells, red blood cells or casts. A cast (an old English word used for worm casts in gardening) is essentially a 'string of beads' of cells. They are an important sign of kidney inflammation.

X-rays, scans, EEG, ECG

Other tests that are not as routine as blood tests and urine, but are important in diagnosis. These include:

- a chest X-ray in a patient with cough or pleurisy
- a brain MRI scan in a patient with lupus or Hughes syndrome who has headache or neurological features
- a kidney scan prior to renal biopsy
- ECG and echocardiography to check the heart.

General treatment of lupus

Introduction

Possibly the most important advance in the treatment of lupus in the past 30 years has been the recognition that things can and do improve, and that medication such as steroids need not be forever!

Key points

- Steroid doses are now lower
- Antimalarials are very useful
- Lifestyle measures are important

Many, perhaps the majority, of my lupus patients ultimately manage on minimal maintenance treatment with low dose Plaquenil® (see Chapter 19) or even no medication at all.

The newer approach to treatment can be summarised as aggressive treatment for severe or acute disease, followed by conservative treatment once the flare is over.

Steroids

These remain the vital medication for acute or active lupus. Usually given as tablets of prednisolone, the dose varies from 5 mg daily up to 30 mg daily or more. The main advantage of steroids is that they are rapidly effective, given the correct dosage. The disadvantages (detailed in Chapter 20) are well known.

Steroids can also be given by injection, for example, either intramuscularly into an inflamed joint or by intravenous drip or pulse injection.

Antimalarials

Widely used in lupus, the quinine family of drugs has been around for over 100 years. The most commonly used drug is hydroxychloroquine (Plaquenil®) and it is particularly effective in the treatment of skin rashes, aches and pains, and fatigue. Plaquenil® is now widely used as a long term maintenance therapy.

Immunosuppressives

Lupus is a disease in which the immune system becomes over-active, and drugs which suppress the immune system have a major role in treatment. The commonly used drugs, described in more detail in Chapter 21, are azathioprine (Imuran®), cyclophosphamide (Cytoxan®), mycophenolate mofetil (Cellcept®) and methotrexate. Newer, targeted drugs (capable of attacking selected components of the immune system) are now coming into use and promise to play an important role in active lupus. One such agent, rituximab (Mabthera®), is reviewed in Chapter 22.

Other drugs

Other medical problems which can arise in lupus patients include raised blood pressure, osteoporosis, depression, headaches, blood clotting, dry eyes, and so on, each of which may require its own specific treatment. One of the advances in our knowledge of lupus has been the recognition of the need to protect against arterial disease (atheroma). Diet, stopping smoking and a more pro-active approach to the treatment of raised cholesterol are all part of lupus management in the 21st century.

Lifestyle

One of the difficulties faced by lupus patients is that they look well. Sometimes others find it hard to understand the fatigue and the fluctuation that are so characteristic of lupus. Most doctors now agree that, once the severe or acute phase is under control, a gradual return to as normal a lifestyle as possible produces the best results. Exercise (within the boundaries of discomfort) is important; indeed, research by my London Lupus Centre colleagues Colin Tench and David D'Cruz showed that graduated exercise programmes actually decreased fatigue scores.

Avoidance of too much direct sunlight (specifically UV light) is wise, and is discussed in Chapter 5.

Allergies

Lupus patients often have a very allergic history, with allergies to antibiotics such as penicillin being common. I have previously reported that allergy to sulphur-containing drugs (notably Septrin®), a sulphur-containing antibiotic, is almost universal. A history of severe Septrin® allergy – 'the septrin provocation test' – is an important clue when taking a history in lupus and Sjögren's patients.

Allergies are also seen to insect bites, certain foods, and sometimes skin contact.

A difficult problem arises with vaccinations and immunisation. For example, some lupus patients experience a flare of disease following flu vaccination. It is hard to give specific advice here. My own advice is to avoid live vaccines if the patient is on high dose steroids or immunosuppressives, but to accept vaccination if there are important reasons to do so, for example if it is strongly recommended when visiting certain countries.

Diet

Is there a diet for lupus? This is probably the most commonly asked question in a lupus clinic. In general, no specific diet has been found to be especially beneficial in lupus, and most patients eat a full and normal diet. Obviously if there are special problems such as raised cholesterol, or fluid retention and raised blood pressure, low fat, low salt diets are indicated.

Having said this, however, there are a number of lupus (and Sjögren's) patients who appear to have clear-cut examples of food allergy, with the aches and pains predictably worsening within 24 hours of certain foods.

While there is no definitive list, common culprits in my clinical experience include gluten-containing foods, red wine, cheese and dairy products. I have had individual patients with adverse reactions, for example, to sodium glutamate, coffee, and shell fish. Unfortunately, there are really no fool-proof tests for such idiosyncrasies, other than experience.

Alternative treatments

In my lupus experience, the majority of patients (over 60% in a recent survey) take various forms of alternative treatment in addition to conventional medicines. I suppose I would do the same.

While the growth of the alternative medicine industry seems unstoppable, and in general is safe, there are two caveats. First, these drugs and treatments are not subjected to the rigorous scrutiny required for conventional medicines. Second, alternative medicine is private medicine and sometimes the financial cost can be a burden.

Family

Lupus is not 'catching' nor is it strongly genetic. So for the woman hoping to have a family, there is no contraindication to pregnancy, providing her health is good (see Chapter 12). It goes without saying that family support is extremely helpful in helping the lupus patient. For this reason above, I believe that education about lupus is critical – for patients and their doctors, friends and supporters.

Where can I find out more?

Chapter 26 lists some of the booklets and websites giving information about lupus. One of our main goals in the London Lupus Centre is to help in this education. We are happy to provide leaflets and information, more details of which can be obtained from our website *www.thelondonlupuscentre.co.uk*.

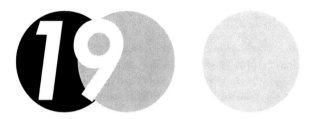

Plaquenil® and antimalarials

Introduction

In 1886, Dr Payne, Consultant at St Thomas' Hospital in London, published a paper indicating that quinine, then widely used for various skin rashes, was also helpful for some of the more general

Key points

- Plaquenil® is safe
- Not damaging to the eyes
- Safe in pregnancy
- Helps fatigue

features of lupus, such as fever, fatigue and joint pains. Quinine, like aspirin, is a 'natural' product derived from the bark of a tree (the South American cinchona tree), and has held an important place in medicine for centuries. Derivatives of quinine (notably chloroquine) were, for many years, the mainstay of treatment for malaria. Unfortunately, chloroquine had some important and limiting side effects, including, importantly, damage to the retina of the eye. Luckily, its successor hydroxychloroquine (trade name Plaquenil®) has proved safe, and is now a mainstay in lupus treatment worldwide.

Properties of Plaquenil®

Plaquenil® usually comes as a standard sized pill (200 mg), most commonly taken once daily. It has a slow action (a long half-life). It can take up to 2 months to start working effectively. Likewise, when stopped, its effects can continue for 1–3 months (see pregnancy). It is well tolerated, rarely causing side effects.

Surprisingly, despite its long history, we still do not know precisely how Plaquenil® works in lupus. It does have a number of properties potentially useful in lupus, including, sun-protection, immunosuppression (mild), anti-clotting (mild) and cholesterol lowering (mild), but these only add up to a part of the picture. When it works, it works well, with the fatigue in many patients clearly improving.

The eye

As chloroquine could damage the retina, there have been many detailed long-term ophthalmic studies of Plaquenil® and the results have been very reassuring. For example, we published a 5 year follow up study with our eye colleagues and found not a single case of retina change in our patients. Indeed, the British Society of Ophthalmology has now published guidelines advising that the previously suggested 6 monthly eye checks are no longer required. Our own practice therefore is to stick to the annual general eye check which our lupus patients undertake routinely.

Side effects

Side effects are rare, the most common being a slightly looser gurgly tummy. Unlike non-steroidal drugs, irritation of the stomach with Plaquenil® is very rare. Long term Plaquenil® use (many months or even years) can, however, produce a slight darkening of the skin and nails though rarely bad enough to stop the drug. Allergic skin reactions are rare; unfortunately they mean stopping the medicine. One side effect on higher doses is blurred vision (lazy eye focusing). Usually seen on a dose of 2 or 3 tablets daily, this naturally frightens the patient who then stops taking the drug. It has nothing to do with retinal damage and is totally reversible.

Dosage

The usual dose is 1 tablet a day (200 mg). In some countries a loading dose of 1 or even 3 tablets a day is given, but I do not follow this practice because of the risk of lazy eye focusing.

Dosage can be varied, for example raising to 2 tablets daily for flares, or reducing to alternate days or even 3 tablets a week for maintenance treatment. Some patients from sunny countries take Plaquenil® in the summer months only.

Pregnancy

We now know that Plaquenil® is safe in pregnancy, both for the mother and the fetus. In the past, many doctors stopped Plaquenil® at the start of pregnancy only to see the expected flare of disease two to three months into the pregnancy. Once the pregnancy is over, it is our standard practice to continue Plaquenil® throughout breast feeding (remember – lupus can flare in the months after pregnancy).

Stopping the drug

An important study from Canada investigated whether women on long term Plaquenil® really needed to take it. In one trial, half the patients stopped taking Plaquenil® and were given a placebo, whie the other half continued taking the drug. The results showed that there were considerably more flares in those who had stopped taking the drug. This is an important observation underlining the important role of Plaquenil® as a maintenance drug in milder lupus.

Quinacrine (Mepacrine®, Atabrine®)

Another antimalarial drug useful in lupus is quinacrine (also called Mepacrine® or Atabrine®). This drug is far less widely used because of two important side effects. First, it has a horrible bitter taste, and second over a period of time it has a tendency to cause some yellowing of the skin. Yet despite these limitations, it has a place in treatment, particularly in severe lupus skin disease. In this situation, I have often used a combination of two antimalarials (eg, Plaquenil® 1 or 2 tablets daily plus Mepacrine® 1 tablet, 100 mg every other day). Although this mixture sounds like cookery I have found it useful, and generally well tolerated.

20

Steroids

Steroids generate very mixed feelings among patients and doctors. There is no doubt that these drugs are of importance in treating lupus, but they are also associated with a number of side-effects. Luckily the side-effects are really only a

Key points

- Steroids are vital in severe lupus
- Lower doses are now used
- Most patients are weaned off
- Intravenous 'pulse' steroids are quick acting

big problem when steroids are used in high doses for a prolonged period of time.

What are steroids?

The name steroid is used to describe a whole class of chemicals produced all the time within the body.

However, when treating lupus we are only interested in the steroids that have anti-inflammatory effects, called the corticosteroids. These steroids reduce inflammation in a number of ways. They reduce the activity of body cells in the immune system, such as the white blood cells, lymphocytes and macrophages. In addition, they reduce the formation of chemicals called cytokines that are used to send messages between white blood cells.

Steroids can be given to treat lupus as tablets, by injection or by infusion into a vein. The most commonly used form is the tablet and this is most often a steroid called prednisolone. Prednisolone can be used in a number of different doses. For mild symptoms of lupus, no steroids may be needed. However, a low dose of 5–7.5 mg per day may be useful. For more serious lupus with kidney involvement, higher doses such as 40–60 mg per day may be used for short periods. In general, thinking has changed over the last 20 years, leading to a reduction in the doses of steroids used.

Steroids may be also given into a vein as an injection or drip. The most commonly used form is methylprednisolone. This way of giving steroids is usually reserved for more serious complications of lupus. In the past, doses of 1,000 mg given daily for three days were used. More recent research suggests that this dose is not always necessary and 500 mg is often adequate.

Side-effects of steroids

Steroids were first used to treat people in the 1950s. They were initially used in patients with severe rheumatoid arthritis. The steroids produced remarkable improvements. This led to a rheumatologist called Hench being awarded the Nobel Prize for medicine. However, after a period of time the patients treated tended to develop a number of side-effects. The most common were weight gain, 'moon-face', high blood pressure, thin bones (osteoporosis), and lowered resistance to infection. Steroids can also change a person's mood, with people largely becoming depressed but also agitated.

Most of the problems associated with steroid use can be reduced by fairly simple measures, including using the lowest possible dose possible for the shortest time. Other medicines may also be used to take the place of steroids. These are called steroid-sparing drugs and include azathioprine and mycophenelate mofetil. Some medicines may be used to protect people from steroid side-effects. These include treatment for thin bones (osteoporosis) in individuals who will need steroids for more than a few weeks. The most common of these bone-protective drugs are bisphosphonates, calcium, and vitamin D.

Summary

Steroids can certainly cause a number of unwanted side-effects. However, using the lowest doses for the shortest possible time has reduced the problems associated with their use. Although care must be taken, steroids remain a vital part of the treatment of lupus, particularly in severe disease.

Immunosuppresives

There are a number of drugs that fall under the general heading of immunosuppressants. However, only a few are widely used in lupus and each is discussed in this chapter.

Azathioprine (Imuran®)

This drug has been used in lupus for over 30 years, and is a tried and trusted agent. Like all the members of this family, it not only suppresses the immune response, but can also affect other dividing cells such as the white blood cells.

Correct dosing is critical, most physicians using 1–2.5 mg per kg body weight daily (usually 100–150 mg daily, occasionally 200 mg). Azathioprine (Imuran®) is widely used firstly in lupus nephritis, and secondly as a steroid sparing agent in patients where it has proved difficult to wean down the steroid dose.

The good news is that for the majority of patients (including, significantly, pregnant patients) azathioprine is well tolerated, with two-monthly blood tests being the only requirement in monitoring.

There are, however, significant problems in some patients. A percentage of individuals (maybe 5% or higher) cannot tolerate the drug. There is almost immediate nausea, and the liver tests become abnormal. We now know that this intolerance is due to the failure to metabolise the drug by an enzyme called tissue inhibitor of metalloproteinases (TIMP). Some units measure this enzyme prior to starting azathioprine, but at present this is not a routine test. Finally, another occasionally very troublesome side effect (especially in kidney transplant patients) is skin warts which can be bad enough to require stopping the drug.

MMF (mycophenolate mofetil/Cellcept®)

Although azathioprine has a long history, its occasionally troublesome side effects, as well as its rather weak profile, has made the search for alternatives a high priority. One agent which promises a great future in lupus is MMF (Cellcept®). This drug, used successfully for many years in the world of organ transplantation, is rapidly coming to the fore as an effective and safe alternative to azathioprine. Early reports tended to concentrate on lupus nephritis, where Cellcept® was shown to be successful in producing disease remission, as well as in maintenance treatment (ongoing treatment). During the past few years, it has gained a place in other aspects of lupus such as muscle disease, low platelets and skin disease.

The tablets are each 500 mg and the usual dose is 3–4 tablets daily (2 g daily). The most common side effect is bowel looseness and occasionally troublesome diarrhoea, which limits the dose. As the drug is newer, there is little data in pregnancy and thus MMF should be stopped prior to pregnancy.

Methotrexate

This is the drug that revolutionised the treatment of rheumatoid arthritis. Its outstanding success in the treatment of inflammatory arthritis has made it a world leader in rheumatic disease. In lupus, however, it has a more limited role, largely because most lupus patients do not have the swollen, inflamed joints suffered by rheumatoid patients.

Methotrexate is used in a small dose usually 7.5 mg weekly, increasing if necessary to 10 mg, 15 mg or higher. It is usual to give the vitamin folic acid once or twice a week as a supplement. Side effects include nausea and mouth ulcers. More serious side effects can be a low blood count and liver abnormalities and a 6 weekly blood count with liver function tests is routine.

Cyclophosphamide (Cytoxan®, Endoxan®)

This is a powerful drug with both good and bad properties. Originally given as a tablet, it was found to be a potent immunosuppressive but because of frequent side effects (nausea, bladder irritation, hair loss), it is now given by intravenous or pulse infusions (together with copious fluids to minimise bladder irritation). For the past three of four decades, most patients with active lupus nephritis have been treated with the 'NIH regimen', a series of weekly then monthly pulses of 1 g of cyclophosphamide, first recommended by doctors at the National Institutes of Health (NIH) in Washington.

This regimen has been largely responsible for the dramatic improvement in outlook in lupus nephritis, with end-stage renal disease and dialysis now being the exception rather than the rule.

The NIH regimen did, however, have major drawbacks; infections (including painful herpes zoster or shingles) developed in 25% of patients, and ovarian failure and infertility in up to 30%, which is totally unacceptable. For this reason, in 1985 I developed a more conservative approach, the so-called 'St Thomas' Hospital regimen'. This generally consisted of 500 mg pulses weekly for 4 weeks, then

500 mg monthly for 3–12 months, after which the milder drug azathioprine (or more recently mofetil) was used.

The results, recently confirmed in a European-wide study (Eurolupus), have been gratifying. The efficiency has been the same, the side effects drastically reduced. For young women with lupus nephritis, the risk of cyclophosphamide-induced infertility has all but vanished.

Other drugs and treatments in lupus

Nonsteroidal anti-inflammatory drugs (NSAIDs)

This is the generic name given to a group of agents used in arthritis. They include such well known drugs as naproxen (Naprosyn®), ibuprofen (Brufen®) and diclofenac (Voltarol®) and newer agents such as etoricoxib (Arcoxia®).

They are useful in those lupus patients with arthritis, and are also used for pleurisy (often in an attempt to reduce the steroid dose). Their main drawback is indigestion, and an increased risk of a stomach ulcer (especially in older people). Also, as they are processed through the kidney, the dose must be carefully monitored in patients with poor renal function.

Thalidomide

This notorious drug, which was found to cause congenital fetal abnormalities if taken in pregnancy, nevertheless has some positive attributes. It has been found to be useful in a number of skin conditions including leprosy, and in the mouth ulcers of AIDS patients. It has also proved useful in some cases of severe skin lupus (especially discoid lupus), dramatically so in some cases. Apart from being restricted to males, and to older females, for whom pregnancy is not an issue, it has another major drawback. While our own studies confirmed its striking success in some cases of resistant skin lupus, it had a tendency to cause neuropathy (mainly severe pins and needles in the feet and hands). New thalidomide derivatives are now being introduced, hopefully without the teratogenicity or the nerve irritation side effects. We await, with hope, their success in lupus treatment.

Dapsone

This drug, used by dermatologists for a variety of skin lesions, is still sometimes used in the treatment of skin lupus. However it can cause anaemia and is rarely the first choice of treatment.

Dihydro-epiandronic acid (DHEA)

This compound, which has very mild male hormone effects, has had something of a cult status as a bringer of youth and is available as an over-the-counter remedy in many countries. Preliminary trials in the US have suggested a beneficial effect in lupus, albeit a mild one. It does have the virtue of having a mild protective effect against osteoporosis. It is not yet officially registered for the treatment of lupus and we await further results.

Rituximab (Mabthera®)

This decade has seen the explosion of new designer drugs. Their names are fairly unpronounceable, but they all end in -mab (short for monoclonal antibody).

Rituximab has been developed by scientists as a magic bullet directed against a specific site on the B cell (the cell which produces the antibodies in SLE and other conditions). And it works! Two injections of Rituximab (also called antiCD20) almost totally abolish B cells. The resultant clinical improvement in lupus has been striking and this new drug is being increasingly tried in patients with very active lupus.

Critically, newer 'sons of rituximab' are already in the pipeline with one called epratuzamab already in clinical trials.

Abatacept (Orencia®)

As scientists become more precise in pinpointing various chemicals involved in inflammation and in cell processing (ie, cells passing on messages to each other), a whole army of antidotes is being generated. One example is abatacept, a drug directed against IL6, which is an important chemical in the inflammation process. Trials of agents such as abatacept are now going on in lupus centres around the world.

Intravenous immunoglobulin (IVIG)

Not exactly a drug, this preparation is simply the pooled antibody (immunoglobulin) of hundreds of healthy donors. The theory is that this 'soup' of antibodies contains antidotes to many of the 'bad' antibodies in lupus and blocks their effect – magic, maybe, but it works, often dramatically. Many sick lupus patients have responded to this 5 day intravenous infusion where other agents had failed.

Unfortunately, IVIG is in very short supply around the world and efforts are underway to purify and concentrate the useful antibodies from the remainder.

Treatment of Hughes syndrome

Anti-clotting drugs

Introduction

Hughes syndrome is often known as sticky blood syndrome. Although not strictly correct, the title is useful as patients who have antiphospholipid antibodies (aPL) in their bloodstream do have a tendency to develop blood clots, in arteries as well as in veins. Logically, therefore, treatment should be with blood-thinning agents which is rather limited at present to aspirin, heparin or warfarin. Medicines aside, there are also lifestyle factors which affect the risk of thrombosis.

> **Key points**
> - Aspirin – milder cases
> - Heparin – useful in acute thrombosis
> - Warfarin - for severe or recurrent clots
> - Newer anticoagulants awaited

General treatment

We are still uncertain of the precise risk figure for thrombosis in an individual positive for aPL, although a number of reports suggest a 50% chance within 10 years if left untreated.

Smoking is certainly an added risk for thrombosis and Hughes syndrome patients are strongly advised to stop. Likewise the oral contraceptive (oestrogen) pill increases the risk, and a number of women with antiphospholipid syndrome (APS) have been found to develop their first clotting problem when starting the pill. Hormone replacement therapy (HRT) in older patients also slightly increases the risk of clotting, though far less than the oral contraceptive pill. Caution is advised in aPL positive women planning HRT, though at present patient risks are weighed up on a case-by-case basis.

Diet may also affect the clotting risk. For example, an interesting study was published by my friend Dr Malawiya, comparing thrombosis risks in aPL positive individuals in India and Kuwait. Thrombotic events were much more common in those patients from Kuwait, which possibly may be due to a less vegetarian diet in this country than in India.

Travel and long haul flights can also add to this risk of thrombosis, and either aspirin or heparin is usually advised, depending on the clinical picture. Finally, aPL positive patients are at a higher risk from thrombosis following surgery. Indeed it is reported that up to 20% of all DVTs are associated with aPL, and that routine pre-operative blood screening for aPL really should be considered.

Aspirin

Like Plaquenil® (which is derived from the cinchona tree), aspirin comes from the bark of a tree (willow tree). It has many beneficial effects, notably in making the platelets of the blood less sticky. Thus it is widely used in cardiology, for example as a preventative measure for recurrent heart attacks.

The usual dose is 75 mg daily (one quarter of an adult aspirin), sometimes 150 mg daily. Side effects such as indigestion on this tiny dose are unusual, with the most common being bruising (evidence that the medicine is doing its job).

Rarely, patients are allergic to aspirin (eg, asthmatics are sometimes worse on the drug) and in this event a very useful (though expensive) aspirin alternative is Plavix® (clopidogrel) 75 mg daily.

Low-dose aspirin is the most widely used medicine in Hughes syndrome. Evidence of its benefits has come from many sources, including pregnancy data in Hughes syndrome where aspirin has contributed significantly to the improved pregnancy and survival figures.

Heparin

For many years, heparin has been the standard first-line treatment for thrombosis. It works quickly and has an excellent safety record. Unfortunately for Hughes syndrome patients, who need long term treatment, it can only be given by injection. However, it is particularly useful in the first half of pregnancy, when warfarin is banned. Most countries now use the newer low molecular weight heparin (eg, Fragmin®, Clexane®), which is easy to self-administer and has far fewer side effects.

Heparin has many uses in APS, for example:

- in patients where warfarin has to be stopped for dentistry or surgery

- in certain APS patients on aspirin who are embarking on long haul flights

- in some Hughes syndrome patients with memory loss or with recurrent migraine attacks.

Warfarin

Warfarin has been in worldwide use for half a century and thousands of patients (eg, those with artificial heart valves) are on lifelong treatment. Apart from its vital property of thinning the blood, warfarin has a remarkably good side effect record (its popular 'rat poison' tag simply being due to its use in high doses to cause bleeding in vermin). Warfarin is (until newer anticoagulants come along) the mainstay of treatment for Hughes syndrome patients with major clotting problems.

The dose varies widely (eg, 3–20 mg daily) with the important measure being the INR, the international normalised ratio – the blood's thickness. The INR is simply a comparison with normal blood. A useful analogy is milk from the supermarket – normal milk has a ratio of 1, half cream a ratio of 2, skimmed milk a ratio of 3 etc.

Patients on warfarin are usually monitored in their local anti-coagulant clinics, where INR is checked and the dosage of warfarin monitored. Most patients with Hughes syndrome seem to need an INR of 2.5 or higher to protect against thrombosis. However patients differ individually: while some patients are symptom-free with an INR of, say, 2.8, in others an INR of 3.4 is needed before the headaches, memory problems and balance disturbances are abolished.

INR self-testing

It is now possible for patients to test their own INR with a simple portable finger-prick machine. A number are on the market, for example the CoaguChek® made by Roche. Just as self-testing for sugar levels has improved the life of millions of diabetics, so also, in my own practice, has INR self-testing improved the quality of life in dozens of my patients. As one patient, a businesswoman, explained, 'It has changed my life, I can travel anywhere without the fear of losing good INR control'.

Many patients face opposition when enquiring about self-testing machines in anticoagulant clinics. In my view this is wrong; after all, it is in the patient's best interests to successfully maintain anticoagulant control.

Other treatment

Steroids

Steroids have proved lifesaving in many diseases, including rheumatoid arthritis and lupus. Their main action is against inflammation. As Hughes syndrome is mainly a clotting disorder rather than an inflammatory disorder, steroids have only limited value.

They do play a major role, however, in those patients with low platelets, as they are effectively the first-line of treatment in acute thrombocytopenia, a rare but dramatic situation in which platelet counts fall (sometimes to less than 5,000).

Steroids are also, of course, used in those patients who have both lupus and APS, especially if there are features of inflammation such as arthritis or pleurisy.

Plasmapheresis (plasma exchange)

In this process, blood from the patient passes into a centrifuge, separating the plasma from the red and white cells. Some thirty years ago we introduced plasma exchange into the treatment of lupus, the hope being that we might be able to separate certain bad components (eg, some antibodies) from the good.

Over the years, the procedure has been somewhat disappointing and not the cure that some had hoped for.

Nevertheless, it is still used in some situations, most commonly in critically ill patients when all other treatments have been tried. In Hughes syndrome a very rare complication is the catastrophic antiphospholipid syndrome, where blood all over the body suddenly seems to coagulate. In this situation, the published data, while sparse, does seem to suggest that a better success rate is seen in those patients undergoing plasmapheresis as part of their management.

Intravenous Immunoglobulin (IVIG)

IVIG comes from the separation of the globulins (antibody containing portion) from pooled blood from hundreds of donors. In this way, it is thought that the product contains antibodies against an army of potential invaders (antigens). Over the years, IVIG has achieved an important niche role both in lupus and in Hughes syndrome. Its major successes have been in the treatment of low platelets, and in the more general treatment of acute flares of disease.

In a sick lupus patient with fever and possible infection where, for example, immunosuppressives might be hazardous, IVIG is often the front line emergency treatment. IVIG has a role in Hughes syndrome when other treatments appear to be failing. It is also sometimes used (safely) in pregnancy.

The downsides of IVIG are its cost and its dosage (requiring an intravenous line for 5 successive days, usually as a hospital inpatient).

Immunosuppressives

To date immunosuppressives (azathioprine, methotrexate, and cyclophosphamide) have been disappointing in Hughes syndrome. Azathioprine (used widely in lupus) also has quite a strong (and troublesome) interaction with warfarin. The newer immunosuppressive MMF has not been adequately tried as yet in Hughes syndrome for any judgement to be made.

One of the newest targeted or 'silver bullet' immunosuppressives, anti-CD20 (Mabthera®, also known as rituximab), has been used in a small number of patients with Hughes syndrome with encouraging results at least in the short term. Watch this space.

New anticoagulants

Everyone treating patients with Hughes syndrome is impatient for the arrival of new anticoagulants, some of which are new tablet versions of heparin, while others are designed to work on other areas of the complicated clotting process.

Unfortunately, one or two have fallen at the last fence, for example, following reports of unexpected side effects in late trials.

Although there is feverish activity in the research world, the truth is, at the time of writing, we are still limited to our old friends – aspirin, heparin, and warfarin.

24

Osteoporosis and lupus

What is osteoporosis?

Osteoporosis is also known as brittle bone disease. This is because individuals with osteoporosis have bones that break (or fracture) more easily than they should. The most common sites for these fractures to occur are in the wrist, spine and hip. The fractures are

Key points

- Brittle bones – fracture risk
- Worse after menopause
- Worse on long term steroids
- Calcium and vitamin D drugs help

painful, but also limit mobility. Not being able to walk around easily leads to a loss of fitness and muscle wasting that can make it difficult for some people to regain independence.

Bones change throughout life

Bones grow and change throughout all our lives. Babies have a skeleton largely made of flexible cartilage, like the cartilage in our noses and ears. Then, as time goes by, we lay down hard bone in the cartilage to form rigid skeleton. The density of this bone is highest in our 20s and 30s, and then starts to reduce slowly. The sex hormone oestrogen is important in maintaining healthy bones, and as its levels decrease after the menopause bones become more fragile. Despite bones becoming thinner after the menopause, the problems of osteoporosis are rarely seen until people reach their 60s or 70s.

Lupus and osteoporosis

People with lupus are more likely to suffer with osteoporosis than their friends of a similar age. Most people with lupus are women, and women never achieve bones that are as dense or strong as those of men. In addition, as women become menopausal, the bone density falls further. Women with lupus may also have an earlier menopause than average. Lupus is associated with inflammation in the blood, and this seems to make bones thinner as well. Being unwell with lupus may also restrict someone's ability to perform exercise or may reduce muscle strength. Regular exercise is important to maintain strong, healthy bones. Finally, many individuals with lupus require treatment with steroids such as prednisolone, and although these medicines may be vital to treatment they can also cause thinning of the bones, making them even more brittle.

All of these factors also lead to a lower bone density and a greater chance of osteoporosis.

How can we detect osteoporosis?

Usually osteoporosis is detected by measuring how strong or dense someone's bones are, or if they have unexpected fracture in the hip, back or wrist. The measurement of bone density is usually done using a machine called a DEXA scanner. It only takes a few minutes to perform the scan, and it does not hurt. The scanner will give a measure of bone density that would allow a diagnosis of osteoporosis to be made.

Osteoporosis is more likely if a patient smokes, drinks alcohol, has a poor diet, does no exercise or takes steroids. Osteoporosis is also more likely if women have an early menopause.

How can we treat osteoporosis?

The first method of treatment is to alter lifestyle by stopping smoking, drinking within the recommended allowance of alcohol per week, eating a good diet and exercising. The diet must contain some calcium and vitamin D. Calcium is found in dairy products and vitamin D is present in vegetables and oily fish. Vitamin D is also made in the skin when it is exposed to sunlight. However, many individuals with lupus have to keep their skin covered to prevent lupus skin rashes or flares of disease. If in doubt it is sensible to consider taking calcium and vitamin D supplements.

If someone is at high risk of getting osteoporosis or has low bone density, a number of treatments can be used. These include giving calcium and vitamin D tablets. There are also a number of medicines that can increase bone strength that can be taken as tablets or injections. The most common of these are medicines called bisphosphonates. To prevent bones getting too thin while someone is taking steroids, bisphosphonate tablets, calcium, and vitamin D are often given at the same time.

Immunology

There have been tangible developments in the understanding of the immune system. Vital molecules that allow immune T cells and B cells to recognise each other, and to protect against predators, are being identified with increasing frequency. These molecules have already played a major part in the development of new drugs such as the anti-CD20 drug rituximab.

Hormones

The clear effect of hormones on lupus is an obvious line for research. For example, can we develop drugs which counteract hormonal effects. The answer so far has been disappointing, but some major research groups are actively working in this field.

Clotting

The major impact of the discovery of the antiphospholipid syndrome on lupus has been referred to in this book. This includes, for example, the use of aspirin, heparin or warfarin for sticky blood where previously high dose steroids might have been used.

There is, however, still a lot to learn. Will there be better drugs than warfarin? What is the mechanism for the thrombosis? Could we block the clot-producing antibodies? Are physicians in affected specialities (eg, orthopaedics, cardiology, surgery, psychiatry) sufficiently updated about the syndrome?

Treatment

New drugs such as mofetil, rituximab and ocrelizumab are emerging in lupus, and, for the first time in my career, many major pharmaceutical companies are investing in lupus treatment research.

25

The future

Lupus has emerged from its cinderella status, and is now the subject of research, international collaboration, conferences and publications. The international journal LUPUS (http://lup.sagepub.com/) published monthly is now in its seventeenth year

Key points

- Advances in genetics
- Advances in immunology
- New drugs at last
- Awareness of lupus improved

and publishes research papers, reviews and letters from colleagues all over the world. Some of the research topics have already been alluded to in this book, and the main ones are summarised here.

Genetics

The developments in genetics in recent years have been spectacular. In the era of the computer, millions of studies relating to the human genome can be carried out in a day. Provided the clinical data fed into these number crunching robots is accurate (an important proviso), it seems likely that the genetic profile leading to a lupus risk will be known before too long. While this information might not lead to a cure, it will be vital for the development of new drugs and vaccines for the prevention and treatment of the disease.

But a somewhat unsung advance may also have had a part to play in the improved outlook in lupus and that is the finer tuning of existing drugs. Steroids, for example, are now routinely tapered down to the lowest clinically effective dose whereas previously they might have been used in far higher doses.

One such example, of which I am personally proud, was my introduction of lower doses of cyclophosphamide in the treatment of lupus nephritis. In 1985, unhappy with the severe side effects of the then widely used regimen (which included infections and ovarian failure) I introduced the 'St Thomas' Hospital regimen' – a standard medium dose regimen of 500 mg cyclophosphamide weekly for 4 weeks, then monthly for 3–9 months. This drastically reduced regimen not only eliminated ovarian failure but was just as effective. Under the leadership of Professor Fred Houssiau in Brussels, this regimen was tested in a European-wide study and convincingly shown to be as effective as the older high dose regimen.

Awareness

Much of the striking improvement in the outcome of lupus comes from factors outside direct treatment of the condition. These include better treatment of infections, raised blood pressure and cholesterol; attention to smoking and other lifestyle issues; and improving healthcare in most poorer countries.

Awareness of lupus is improving, with many countries having active patient support groups. Yet it is still surprising that lupus (more common than multiple sclerosis or leukaemia) is as yet unknown to much of the population.

Why don't lupus patients catch colds?

Lastly, as a clinician, I believe that this old fashioned clinical observation has an important part to play in advancing research into the disease and its treatment.

Treating large numbers of patients with a particular disease over a long period of time can lead to useful clinical observations (which then of course need to be verified). For example, it has been my experience that lupus patients seem to catch fewer colds than their spouses or relatives. Might this be due to steroids or to the active immune system? It is also my strong impression that malignancy is less common in lupus patients (this subject has been confused in the past because of the inclusion of Sjögren's syndrome, which is associated with an increased risk of non-Hodgkin's lymphoma).

And why are lupus patients so sensitive to mosquito and other insect bites? And are food allergies truly more common in lupus patients?

All these and other clinical impressions need proving or disproving in carefully planned studies. However, I hope that they make a point – that basic clinical observations by patients and doctors can and do contribute in the battle to improve knowledge of this disease. And in so doing, they may just help to improve the lupus patient's lot.

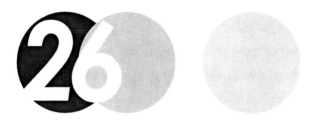

Where can I find out more?

Patient books

- Hughes G. Lupus: the facts. Oxford: Oxford University Press, 2000.

- Hughes G. Hughes syndrome: a patient's guide. London: Springer, 2001.

- Norton Y (ed.). Lupus: a GP guide to diagnosis. London: Lupus UK, 2000.

Textbooks

- Lahita R (ed.) Systemic lupus erythematosus, 4th edition. San Diego: Academic Press, 2004.

- Wallace D & Hahn B (ed.) Dubois' lupus erythematosus, 5th edition. Philadelphia: Lippincott Williams & Wilkins, 1997.

- Khamashta M (ed.) Hughes syndrome: antiphospholipid syndrome, 2nd edition. London: Springer, 2006.

Charities & websites

- St Thomas' Lupus Trust (www.lupus.org.uk)

- Hughes Syndrome Foundation (www.hughes-syndrome.org)

- Lupus UK (www.lupusuk.org.uk)

- The London Lupus Centre (www.thelondonlupuscentre.co.uk)

Journals

- LUPUS. An International Journal (Sage Publications) (http://lup.sagepub.com)